Clinical Otology and Audiology

Second Edition

G. G. Browning, MB, ChB, MD, FRCS (Edin), FRCS (Glas)
Professor of Otolaryngology, University of Glasgow, UK
Consultant Otolaryngologist, Department of Otolaryngology and Head and Neck Surgery,
Royal Infirmary, Glasgow, UK
Consultant Otologist, MRC Institute of Hearing Research (Scottish Section), Royal Infirmary,
Glasgow, UK
Senior Clinical Adviser, MRC Institute of Hearing Research, Nottingham, UK

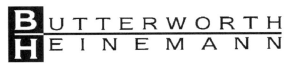

OXFORD BOSTON JOHANNESBURG MELBOURNE NEW DELHI SINGAPORE

For Annette, all the Gs and a J

Butterworth-Heinemann
Linacre House, Jordan Hill, Oxford OX2 8DP
225 Wildwood Avenue, Woburn, MA 01801-2041
A division of Reed Educational and Professional Publishing Ltd

ℛ A member of the Reed Elsevier plc group

First published 1986
Second edition 1998

British Library Cataloguing in Publication Data
A catalogue record for this book is available from the British Library

Library of Congress Cataloguing in Publication Data
A catalogue record for this book is available from the Library of Congress

ISBN 0 7506 3373 5

Typeset by Keytec Typesetting Ltd., Bridport, Dorset
Printed and bound in Great Britain by the Bath Press, Somerset

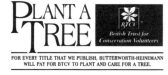

FOR EVERY TITLE THAT WE PUBLISH, BUTTERWORTH-HEINEMANN
WILL PAY FOR BTCV TO PLANT AND CARE FOR A TREE.

Contents

Preface to second edition

Copies of the first edition of *Clinical Otology and Audiology* have become impossible to procure. Second-hand copies rarely come on the market and library copies have inevitably 'gone astray'. This text is particularly in demand for pre-examination reading and photocopying is common. Hence, it seemed appropriate to produce a second edition.

A new edition rather than a revision was required because of the considerable technical advances there have been since 1986 when the first edition was published, such as cochlear implants, bone-anchored hearing aids, otoacoustic emissions and magnetic resonance imaging. The need for a new edition became even more evident once writing began. For example, there have been considerable changes in our attitude to the psychosocial aspects of vertigo and tinnitus with an increasing emphasis on counselling. Hearing aids have become increasingly smaller, with a greater range of acoustical options. Real ear measures of hearing aid gain greatly increase the ability to tailor this to the pure tone audiogram and computerized methods are available to estimate likely benefit. The methods of assessment of benefit from management, either by medicines, surgery or aids, have improved as has our understanding of how to rate disability and measure the resultant quality of life.

This edition includes the paediatric aspects of otology and audiology as this was felt to be a deficiency that could not be rectified by reading other texts. Involvement with the MRC-funded multicentre Trial of Alternative Regimes of Glue Ear Treatment (Target) has given me access to as yet unpublished data which is referenced as MRC Target data.

Preface to first edition

Considering the number of otological and audiological textbooks that are available why is it considered necessary to write yet another? The answer is that none of them has been written in the form of a practical guide to help otolaryngologists diagnose, investigate and manage patients with ear conditions. Most texts are primarily discussions of the aetiology and the results of investigations and of management of various conditions, but give little guidance as to how to arrive at the diagnosis and of how the audiological tests might help to do so. In addition the number of pages devoted to a specific condition is by no means related to its incidence in an otolaryngological clinic. Because of this it is not uncommon for trainees to consider that the two commonest causes of a sensorineural hearing impairment are Ménière's syndrome and acoustic neuroma. The amount that is written about a subject is usually proportional to the surgical interest but on the other hand it is difficult to write extensively about something, no matter how common it is, if there is nothing known about it or little one can do for it. So the intellectual emphasis, but not necessarily the number of pages in this text, is devoted to how the average otolaryngologist might investigate and manage patients with the commoner hearing disorders.

Most of the data presented are based on the otology and audiology practice at Glasgow Royal Infirmary (GRI data). Numerous clinical reports have emanated from this practice over the years, often in association with the Scottish Section of the Medical Research Council's Institute of Hearing Research (MRC IHR) which is also based at the Royal Infirmary. In the analysis of the clinical and audiometric data a scientific approach has been taken and a similar approach has been taken with the data reported from other centres. However, there is still a considerable amount of art in the practice of medicine and it is incorrect to think that science, and in this case audiology, has all the answers. It is natural that those offering such a service are more enthusiastic about its role than the facts merit. If the roles of both otology and audiology are critically evaluated it is inevitable that, in many instances, they will be less accurate than they are often portrayed. Many questions remain to be answered by properly conducted, prospective, clinical studies but until these have been reported, patients will still have to be seen, investigated and managed. The approach that is suggested is only one of many possible alternatives and, though it is unlikely to become universally accepted, it should at least make the reader examine more critically his own current techniques.

Acknowledgements

As before, Professor Stuart Gatehouse and Mr Iain R.C. Swan at the Scottish Section of the MRC Institute of Hearing Research (IHR) have been extremely helpful in commenting upon drafts. My research involvement with them and with other colleagues, particularly at the MRC IHR Headquarters in Nottingham, has, I hope, added to knowledge but also increased my understanding of the problems that occur at the interface between otology and audiology.

Nancy Donald who typed the manuscript and Carol Fulton who helped considerably with the audiograms and other figures are thanked.

G.G.B.

1 Hearing

Hearing is perhaps man's most important sense, for without it his power to communicate is greatly diminished. It is, after all, this superior ability to communicate that sets man above other animals. Unfortunately it is frequently affected by disease so that a patient develops a hearing impairment which results in a hearing disability.

As this stepwise concept is basic to the investigation and management of patients with hearing disorders it is worth explaining in greater detail. An organ may be affected by a disease or it may be injured or removed. Whether this is evident or not often depends on whether the function of the organ is sufficiently deranged to cause impairment. Whether this then gives rise to any disability depends on factors apart from the degree of impairment, such as the need for the function and the ability to compensate for the impairment.

In the case of the auditory system, patients frequently present with a hearing impairment and otolaryngologists usually devote most of their attention to identifying the site affected and the pathology responsible. Though this is important, it is equally important to assess the resultant disability because at present there is no specific therapy for most of the pathological conditions that affect the auditory system, the exception being some of those that affect the middle ear. As such, in most instances the management is of the disability rather than of the disease. Unfortunately, methods of assessing the former tend to have been neglected which makes it difficult to gauge the relative benefits of medication, surgery and the provision of a hearing aid in relieving disability.

Ear disease

Pathology can affect any anatomical part of the auditory pathway (*Figure 1.1*), singly or in combination. When in combination, it can be because of spread of the pathology, usually a middle ear inflammatory process spreading to the inner or outer ear. Alternatively, when a neurological part is affected, this can have a secondary pathological effect on the connections to that part. Thus, loss of hair cells in the inner ear leads to secondary degeneration in the auditory nerve.

Ear pathology may or may not be symptomatic. Post-mortem temporal bone histology frequently identifies otosclerotic foci or acoustic neuromas that were clinically silent. However, with these two exceptions the majority of ear pathology is symptomatic. History-taking of symptoms has the dual objective of helping identify the pathology and of assessing the associated disability (see p. 5). In those with ear pathology, hearing impairment is the commonest and usually the most dominant symptom.

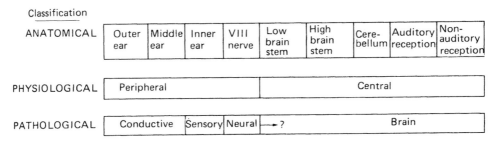

Classification

ANATOMICAL	Outer ear	Middle ear	Inner ear	VIII nerve	Low brain stem	High brain stem	Cere-bellum	Auditory reception	Non-auditory reception

PHYSIOLOGICAL	Peripheral	Central

PATHOLOGICAL	Conductive	Sensory	Neural → ?	Brain

Figure 1.1 Auditory pathway

Hearing impairment

Audiometry is the main method of assessing the hearing. Pure tone audiometry, or less frequently speech audiometry, is used to determine the degree of impairment (*Table 1.1*), and the site and type of the impairment (*Figure 1.1*). A conductive impairment is due to pathology in the external, middle or inner ear, and primarily attenuates sound in terms of its loudness. A sensory impairment is due to pathology in the inner ear, most commonly loss of hair cells and, apart from attenuating the loudness of the sound, there is often a loss of frequency discrimination and timing (temporal) abilities. Clinically and audiometrically, there may be evidence of recruitment, when sounds can appear abnormally loud. A neural impairment is due to pathology in the cochlear division of the eighth cranial nerve and, because it can affect both the afferent and efferent nerve fibres, has the same effect as a sensory impairment. The clinical distinction between a sensory and a neural impairment can be important, particularly in the diagnosis of acoustic neuroma (see p. 61) which affect the cochlear nerve. Unfortunately many of the behavioural audiometric tests that attempt to make this distinction, such as alternate loudness balance, cannot do it accurately mainly because a sensory impairment is almost invariably accompanied by a neural impairment because of secondary, retrograde degeneration of the nerve. This also applies the other way round, in that cochlear nerve pathology causes secondary hair cell loss. Hence, sensorineural impairments are the norm.

Central impairments are caused by pathology in the brain stem or higher audiological centres where the afferent neurological input from both ears is processed for localization and interpretation of the sounds. Audiometric assessment of this central processing is difficult and primarily of interest in research rather than in a clinical context.

Table 1.1 Classification system used in this text to describe the severity of a hearing impairment (the pure tone averages are based on those at 0.5, 1, 2 and 4 kHz)

Pure tone average (dB)	Severity
0–24	Normal
25–50	Mild
51–70	Moderate
71–90	Severe
91–110	Profound
110+	Total

Prevalence

Ascertaining the prevalence of hearing impairment in the population has to take into account the fact that man has two ears. When the prevalence of pathology is being looked at, it is usual to take it as the percentage of individuals with a disease in one or both ears, with the ratio of the population with unilateral as opposed to bilateral disease being stated. Ascertaining the prevalence of hearing impairment can be done in a similar manner, once what constitutes a hearing impairment has been defined. This is usually taken from the four frequency average of the pure tone thresholds over 0.5, 1, 2 and 4 kHz, though sometimes for conduction impairments a three frequency average over 0.5, 1 and 2 kHz is used, and for noise trauma a three frequency average over 1, 2 and 3 kHz is used. The average that defines an impairment is usually taken as 25 or 30 dB HL (Hearing Level).

It is also possible to state the prevalence of different degrees of impairment using a classification such as in *Table 1.1*. Using such systems can lead to misinterpretation because the terms used for degrees of impairment are the same as those used for degrees of disability. However they are used in different ways. Thus, an individual with a profound impairment in one and normal hearing in the other ear is not profoundly deaf as disability is primarily determined by the hearing in the better hearing ear (see below).

The prevalence of hearing impairment needs to be known for the better and poorer hearing ears. *Table 1.2* shows the prevalence of hearing impairment in the adult British population as assessed in the MRC National Study of Hearing (Davis, 1989; Browning and Gatehouse, 1992; Davis, 1995). Overall 14 per cent have an impairment of 25 dB HL or poorer in their better ear, but this increases to 42 per cent in those over the age of 60 years. Impairments are commoner in men and those in manual occupations. Overall sensorineural impairments are more common than conductive impairments when defined as an air–bone gap of 15 dB or greater over 0.5, 1 and 2 kHz. Conductive impairments constitute a higher proportion in the poorer hearing ear and in the young. Prevalence data for children are given in Chapter 12.

Table 1.2 Population prevalence (per cent) in adults of a hearing impairment* in the better and poorer hearing ears, overall and in 20-year age bands, broken down into sex and occupational groups and with the ratio of sensorineural (SN) to conductive (CON) impairments

	Prevalence in better ear	SN/CON ratio	Prevalence in poorer ear	SN/CON ratio
Overall	14 (13–15)	6.5:1	18 (16–19)	2:1
Age (years):				
18–40	1.5 (1–3)	4:1	3.5 (2–5)	1:1
41–60	11 (9–13)	4:1	17 (15–20)	2:1
61–80	42 (38–46)	11:1	45 (41–50)	3:1
Sex:				
Women	12 (10.5–14)	5:1	15 (13–17)	2:1
Men	16 (14–17)	8:1	21 (19–23)	2.5:1
Occupational group:				
Non-manual	12 (11–14)	7:1	17 (15–19)	3:1
Manual	15 (13–17)	6:1	19 (17–21)	2:1

*A hearing impairment is defined as a pure tone threshold averaged over 0.5, 1, 2 and 4 kHz of 25 dB HL or poorer. The 95% confidence limits are given in parentheses (after Browning and Gatehouse, 1992)

Hearing disability

In most circumstances a patient's hearing disability is determined by the hearing in their better hearing ear. This is because sound, even though presented on the poorer side, will be heard by the better ear because sound can go round the skull, albeit attenuated in its loudness (*Figure 1.2*). The amount of attenuation varies with frequency (*Table 2.2*, p. 7) but for the speech frequencies it is usually taken as −15 dB. Thus a patient totally deaf in one ear but with normal hearing in the other, will hear a speaker on their dead ear side at 65 − 15 = 50 dB A which is sufficiently loud for it to be comprehended (*Figure 1.3*).

Thus, if one wishes to know the population

Table 1.3 UK adult population prevalence (per cent) of hearing impairment in the better hearing ear, together with the percentage of those with a hearing aid in each impairment category

Pure tone average (dB HL)	Population prevalence	Cumulative prevalence	Possess aid
< 25	84.0	84	0.2
25–29	4.9	89	1.4
30–34	3.0	92	6.6
35–39	2.4	94	9.3
40–44	1.9	96	18.6
45–54	1.8	98	37.2
55–64	1.0	99	57.3
65+	1.0	100	88.6

(After Davis, 1997)

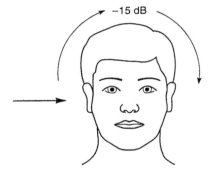

Figure 1.2 Average transcranial attenuation of free-field sound in a quiet environment

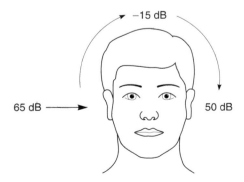

Figure 1.3 Example of transcranial attenuation

prevalence of hearing impaired individuals the prevalence of hearing impairment in the better ear is looked at. In these circumstances it is useful to grade the severity of the impairment because the main use of such data is for policy making (*Table 1.3*). Thus, one might want to know the population prevalence of total hearing impairment to plan a cochlear implant service. If one wishes to know the prevalence in the population to determine the needs for hearing aids, the majority of individuals do not seek advice until their thresholds are greater than 45 dB HL (*Lancet* Editorial, 1987) even though an individual with a 25 dB HL threshold in their better hearing ear would benefit from a hearing aid. Two per cent have an impairment greater than 45 dB HL in their better hearing ear which is thus the relevant figure to take rather than the prevalence of hearing impairment worse than 25 dB HL in the poorer ear (*Table 1.3*).

Further reading

Davis, A.G. (1997). Epidemiology. In *Adult Audiology*, Vol. 2, Chap. 3, Scott-Brown's Otolaryngology, 6th Edition, Butterworth-Heinemann, Oxford.

2 Clinical assessment

The clinical assessment of a patient with otological symptoms has three inter-related components: the history, otoscopy and the assessment of hearing. Sometimes, in addition, examination of the nose, post-nasal space and balance are indicated. This chapter deals with the history, otoscopy and hearing assessment in an adult whose main complaint is hearing impairment.

The history

In medicine, history taking can be helpful in three main ways:

- it can help to diagnose a disease;
- it can assess the patient's symptoms and consequent disability; and
- options can then be formulated alongside a knowledge of what has already been tried.

Because of our ability to diagnose the majority of external and middle ear conditions by otoscopy, the history is often of little additional value in coming to a diagnosis. Thus, in a patient with otoscopic evidence of chronic otitis media, the object of taking a history is not to make the diagnosis but to assess the resultant disability and to plan management. Equally, if an audiogram is available when a patient is seen, history taking is very different in those with a sensorineural as opposed to a conductive impairment. The temptation then is not to carry out the clinical assessment in the traditional order of history followed by examination.

Indeed, the order of partial history, followed by examination, including audiometry, followed by further history has much to commend it.

The history in diagnosis

Table 2.1 is a list of the commoner otological conditions with those that can be diagnosed by otoscopy being asterisked. They comprise the majority of external and middle ear conditions. Inner ear conditions are mainly diagnosed from the history, sometimes backed up by investigation. How a specific diagnosis is made is discussed in more detail in Chapters 4, 5, 6 and 7.

The history in disability assessment

The fact that a symptom is present does not mean that all patients have a similar disability.

Table 2.1 Main method of diagnosis

Commoner otological conditions	Main method of diagnosis	
	History	Otoscopy
Wax		*
Otitis externa		*
Acute otitis media		*
Otitis media with effusion		*
Chronic otitis media		*
Otosclerosis	*	
Traumatic ossicular disruption	*	
Sensorineural impairment:	*	
Age related	*	
Noise trauma	*	
Drugs	*	
Head injury	*	
Acoustic neuroma		
Vestibular syndromes	*	

This is particularly obvious in patients with a hearing impairment where the degree and symmetry of the loss, along with the patient's lifestyle and motivation, combine to give different degrees of disability. With symptoms such as ear discharge the factors which contribute to the disability are less recognized but psychosocial factors have a considerable impact. A fuller discussion of how to assess hearing disability is left to Chapters 9 and 10 but it is important to realize that the disability is usually what determines management rather than the symptoms *per se*.

The history in deciding management

Knowledge of previous management and of what benefit it has been helps to clarify future management options. Thus, previous surgery considerably affects the decision as to how to proceed in those with a conductive impairment.

Otoscopy

How to perform otoscopy and interpret the findings would take a whole textbook to explain (see, for example, Wormald and Browning, 1996) and will not be attempted here. Suffice to say that the likely otoscopic diagnosis varies with the patient's age and symptoms. Thus, a young adult with a hearing impairment is more likely to have chronic otitis media than a sensorineural impairment, whilst an elderly patient is more likely to have a sensorineural impairment than chronic otitis media, though he/she may have both.

Removal of wax to visualize the tympanic membrane is mandatory if there is a conductive impairment so that an otoscopic diagnosis can be made. The exception to this is children in whom otitis media with effusion is likely. In this situation tympanometry can be of diagnostic value and can be carried out in the presence of wax (see p. 138).

Clinical masking of hearing

In clinical testing of hearing it is important to mask out hearing in the non-test ear. The rules and methods involved are different from those in audiometry.

Air conduction masking

Sounds arriving via air at the ear on one side will also be heard by the ear on the other side, but because of the head shadow they will be attenuated by an amount depending on the frequency (*Table 2.2*). As the minimum attenuation at the lower frequencies is 0 dB and as it is wiser to mask unnecessarily than to omit masking when necessary, the rule is that the non-test ear should always be masked when clinically testing by air conduction. The same rule does not apply in audiometry.

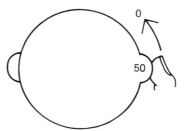

Figure 2.1 Effective masking level (dB) of tragal rubbing

Methods

Unfortunately there is no single method that can produce the required range of masking sound levels, so no one method is suitable for all situations (Table 2.3). For example, there will be occasions when tragal rubbing provides insufficient masking. On the other hand, in most circumstances a Barany box will produce too much masking and will mask the test ear as well as the non-test ear. There are three commonly used methods.

Tragal rubbing

Occluding the external auditory canal by putting a finger on the tragus only attenuates sounds by ~ 10 dB (Hinchcliffe, 1955) and so is of no value. On the other hand, if the tragus is rubbed at the same time (*Figure 2.1*), speech will be attenuated by ~ 50 dB (Swan, 1984).

Table 2.2 Amount (dB) the head shadow attenuates sound coming via air from the contralateral ear

	Frequency (kHz)						
	0.25	*0.5*	*1*	*2*	*3*	*4*	*8*
Mean	1	1	1	7	10	13	10
Maximum	2	4	5	11	15	18	15
Minimum	0	0	0	5	9	10	5

(After Shaw, 1974)

Table 2.3 Appropriate method of masking the non-test ear when voice testing

Whispered voice	At 2 feet	Tragal rubbing
Whispered voice	At 6 inches	Tragal rubbing
Conversational voice	At 2 feet	Tragal rubbing
Conversational voice	At 6 inches	Tragal rubbing
Loud voice		Barany box

The advantage of tragal rubbing over other methods is that the masking sound is produced within the external auditory canal and there is no risk of the sound crossing over and masking the test ear. However, there is a danger of undermasking if the speech is louder than 70 dB A. This means that a Barany box will be necessary when using a loud voice in free-field speech testing. Tragal rubbing will also be insufficient when using tuning forks in those with a severe or profound loss, but in these circumstances the tests are hard to interpret because it is difficult to activate the tuning forks sufficiently for them to be heard.

Paper rubbing

Continuously rubbing a piece of paper between the thumb and index finger produces a consistent broad-band sound. It does not matter what type of paper is used but rubbing the fingers without paper is insufficiently loud for any practical purpose.

Barany box

For many years a Barany noise-box was the standard method of clinical masking. This produces a broad-band noise although there can be marked dips in the frequency spectrum of some boxes and the noise can be irregular. The maximum sound output varies from box to box but a lower limit of 90 dB A can be assumed when a box is held at right angles to the ear and 100 dB A when held over the ear (*Figure 2.2*). These levels are sufficient to mask in all practical circumstances but there is a danger that, because the sound can travel round the skull to the test ear, this will be masked as well (*Figure 2.3*). Eighty per cent of normal ears will be masked by a Barany box in the other ear as evidenced by the inability to

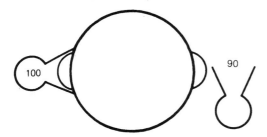

Figure 2.2 Effective masking level (dB) of a Barany box held over (100 dB A) and held at right angles to the ear (90 dB A) (after Swan, 1984)

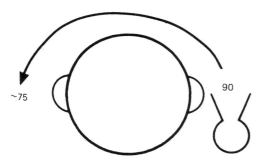

Figure 2.3 Potential level (dB) of cross-masking that can occur with a Barany box

detect a whispered voice at 2 feet (Swan, 1984). Because of this a Barany box should only be used in free-field speech testing when

testing an ear with a severe or profound impairment, i.e. one that cannot hear a conversational voice at 6 inches (see below).

Bone conduction masking

With bone conduction, the transcranial attenuation from one ear to the other is taken as zero (*Figure 2.4*). So in theory, when performing tuning fork tests, the bone conduction should always be masked, but in practice this can be difficult. A Barany box will be necessary as tragal and paper rubbing will provide insufficient bone conduction masking when a conductive impairment is present.

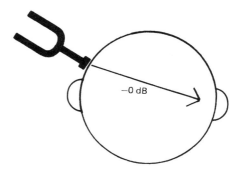

Figure 2.4 Transcranial attenuation of bone conduction

Free-field voice tests of hearing

It is remarkable how often clinicians omit to assess a patient's hearing by free-field voice tests. Assessments often done are the Rinne and Weber tuning fork tests which aim to determine whether an impairment is conductive or sensorineural. How tuning fork tests can be interpreted in the absence of knowledge of the degree of impairment is a mystery. Free-field voice testing takes only 1–2 minutes and, though not as reliable as pure tone or speech audiometry, is of value for the following reasons.

• Audiometry may not be needed: There are

two common circumstances where audiometry may be dispensed with as a result of free-field voice testing. The first is where a previous audiogram is available and there has been no change in symptoms. The second is where screening of the hearing is required. This can be in patients without otological symptoms, such as the elderly, or in those who require reassurance that their hearing is normal.

• As a check on audiometry: Following otoscopy and free-field voice testing, supplemented by Rinne tests where indicated, it should be possible to predict the type and severity of the impairment in each ear. Comparison can then be made with the audiogram and, where discrepancies arise, one or both must be incorrect. Exaggerating thresholds when claiming compensation for noise trauma is the commonest reason for them both to be wrong (Chapter 8). Apart from this, another common reason is difficulty with masking. This occurs most frequently in those with a conductive or asymmetric impairment where it is important to have accurate results.

Method

Free-field voice testing is primarily a method of detecting whether a hearing impairment is present in one or both ears and, whichever is the case, to determine its severity. This is achieved by assessing the threshold for speech by varying the vocal effort and the distance from the ear to produce a range of sound levels of speech.

It is first explained to the patient that they are expected to repeat back, as accurately as possible, what they hear being said by the examiner. The examiner then stands behind the patient to obviate speech reading and says a test word loudly enough to ensure that the task is understood. Thereafter, combinations of numbers and letters (5 B 3) are used as this gives a large variety of combinations. Bisyllable words (e.g. cowboy, football) are often used for children. It is normal to test the better hearing ear first if there is one. The non-test ear is masked by tragal rubbing. The patient's free-field threshold is the voice and distance level at which they get more than 50 per cent correct. It is usual to assess the thresholds by gradually increasing the relative loudness of the voice, so that the examiner starts using a whispered voice 2 feet (60 cm) away from the patient, which is the furthest away he can reach when masking the non-test ear. Provided a whisper is used, and this is best achieved by exhaling first, a patient who does not hear a whispered voice at arm's length is hearing impaired, that is, would benefit from amplification (pure tone average (PTA) ⩾ 25 dB HL). If the patient can repeat this back this does not actually mean that the hearing is normal, as a normal hearing ear will hear a whisper at least 12 feet (4 m) away. Rather it

means that the likely associated disability is insufficient to merit management.

If the patient fails to hear a whispered voice at 2 feet the relative sound level is increased in steps to a whispered voice at 6 inches (15 cm), to a conversational voice at 2 feet, to a conversational voice at 6 inches, to a loud voice at 2 feet and finally to a loud voice at 6 inches. For each new presentation, the number/letter combinations should be changed to avoid the patient recognizing them from previous presentations. The test is terminated when a patient repeats 50 per cent of the words correctly at any one voice and distance level. When using a loud voice, a Barany box must be used as tragal rubbing provides insufficient masking. If there is any doubt concerning a threshold, the examiner can test again at a lower voice level.

Clinical voice tests have been criticized because the sound level of speech varies between examiners and there is a considerable difference in the sound levels that are produced by an examiner on different occasions, particularly in whispering. To avoid this, whispering should be done after full expiration.

Despite the above criticisms, in the hands of experienced otologists, monaural, free-field speech can reliably screen individuals for a hearing impairment greater than 25 dB HL and can grade the severity of a hearing impairment into normal, mild/moderate and severe/profound.

Interpretation

Screening for hearing impairments

Individuals with a speech frequency average greater than 30 dB HL will be unable to hear a whispered voice 2 feet from the test ear. The sensitivity ('hit rate') of this is 95 per cent and the false-positive rate 10 per cent (*Table 2.4*). Hence, if a patient can hear a whispered voice 2 feet from his ear the clinician can be fairly certain that the pure tone thresholds will be better than 30 dB HL and in many instances this will make an audiometric evaluation unnecessary.

Grading the severity of an impairment

A comparison is made in *Table 2.5* of the free-field thresholds against the mean pure tone

Table 2.4 Sensitivity and specificity of a hearing impairment being detected by an individual's inability to hear a whispered voice at 2 feet

	Percentage	
Impairment	Sensitivity	Specificity
PTA over 0.5, 1 and 2 kHz:		
≤ 25 dB HL	86	94
≤ 30 dB HL	95	90
≤ 35 dB HL	100	84
PTA over 0.5, 1 and 2, 4 kHz:		
≤ 25 dB HL	91	96
≤ 30 dB HL	96	91
≤ 35 dB HL	98	86

(After Browning *et al.*, 1989)

Table 2.5 Comparison of free-field voice thresholds and pure tone average (PTA) over 0.5, 1, 2 and 4 kHz

		PTA		
		Mean	Percentiles	
Voice level	Distance	(dB)	5th	95th
Whisper	2 feet	12	–	27
	6 inches	34	20	47
Conversation	2 feet	48	38	60
	6 inches	56	48	67
Loud	2 feet	76	67	87

(After Swan and Browning, 1985)

average (PTA; p. 27) in 200 ears, along with the 5th and 95th percentiles (Swan and Browning, 1985). Though there is some overlap, patients can be divided into three groups by free-field voice testing: PTA less than 30 dB HL; PTA 30–70 dB HL; and PTA greater than 70 dB HL. This corresponds to normal, mild/moderate and severe/profound impairments, respectively.

Rinne test

The Rinne test is the most frequently used tuning fork test, its stated role being to identify a conductive defect. It is extremely helpful to have performed free-field voice testing prior to doing the Rinne test, because knowledge of the degree of impairment and the symmetry between ears greatly aids interpretation. Thus if there is gross asymmetry, there is the possibility of a false-negative Rinne (see below). Such knowledge is also of benefit in deciding how to mask. Thus a Barany box is necessary in a patient with a unilateral severe impairment.

Method

The correct method of performing the Rinne test is well described elsewhere (Hinchcliffe, 1981) but some practical points are worth making. Forks of 512 Hz are usually preferred but there is evidence (Doyle *et al.*, 1984; Browning and Swan, 1988) that a 256 Hz fork is more accurate. There is the potential problem that forks with a frequency lower than 256 Hz

can make it difficult for a patient to distinguish between hearing the sound and feeling it by vibration. It is difficult to sufficiently activate forks with a frequency higher than 512 Hz for them to be heard by those with a moderate or severe sensorineural impairment.

The tuning forks should be as heavy as possible, as the sound level produced by light forks decays rapidly. This is a disadvantage as there is inevitably a time delay between asking the patient to compare the air and the bone conduction. Though forks vary, a decay of 10 dB every 10 seconds is the slowest that can be anticipated.

Activating a 512 Hz fork by compressing the tines between the fingers produces a sound level of ∼ 70 dB SPL (sound pressure level) whereas hitting it against a knee or elbow, without causing pain, produces a sound level of ∼ 90 dB SPL.

When testing air conduction, the tines of the fork should be held directly in line with the external auditory canal, as holding it at an angle diminishes the sound level.

In testing bone conduction, it is important to

make good contact with the skull. This is not achievable on the mastoid tip, the best position being on the flat bone just superior and posterior to the external canal. It is also important that firm pressure is used because the sound level can vary by as much as 15 dB with different degrees of pressure. As the patient's head tends to move away from the tuning fork, it is best to hold the head steady on the contralateral side using the examiner's free hand.

The patient can be asked to make a comparison between the relative loudness of the air and the bone conduction. Alternatively, the sound in one of the test modes can be allowed to decay until it is no longer heard and the patient is then asked if they can hear it by the other mode. In general, loudness comparison techniques identify smaller air–bone gaps than decay methods (Golabek and Stephens, 1979; Browning and Swan, 1988). By convention the results are reported as Rinne positive when the air conduction is louder than the bone conduction and Rinne negative when the bone conduction is louder than the air conduction. Many, including the author, find it difficult to remember which is which, so reporting the results as to which route is louder bypasses this problem.

False-negative results

It is theoretically important to mask the non-test ear whenever the bone conduction is being tested, particularly when testing the poorer hearing ear. This is because the bone conduction on the poorer hearing side may be heard by the other, better ear and give a false-negative Rinne. The only way to mask the bone conduction is by making a sound at the external auditory meatus in the non-test ear. If there is a hearing impairment in the non-test ear, tragal rubbing (*Figure 2.1*) and even a Barany box (*Figure 2.2*) may be insufficiently loud. If a Barany box was used routinely there would be a considerable danger of masking the bone conduction in the test ear as well (*Figure 2.3*). Knowledge of the degree of impairment by free-field voice testing helps decide which method to use, but even then there is often some uncertainty. Because of this, many otologists omit to mask tuning fork tests unless there is gross asymmetry in the hearing.

Validity

It is generally held that the Rinne test will reliably detect a conductive defect of 20 dB or greater. This is not so! This is the level at which 50 per cent of patients with an air–bone gap of 20 dB will be Rinne positive and 50 per cent will be Rinne negative (Crowley and Kaufman, 1966; Golabek and Stephens, 1979; Browning and Swan, 1988).

The value of the Rinne test is best evaluated on data which has analysed the proportion of ears with different sizes of air–bone gap which are Rinne positive and negative. The false-negative and false-positive diagnosis rates can then be calculated for each size of air–bone gap. An example of such an analysis is shown in *Figure 2.5*. From this and other studies it is possible to calculate (*Table 2.6*) the size of air–bone gap that will be correctly identified 50, 75 and 90 per cent of the time, the first value being included as this is the size of air–bone gap that would be correctly detected at the same level by tossing a coin. Though each of the studies can be criticized in different ways, the overall conclusion is inescapable: the Rinne test will *not* reliably detect (i.e. on 90% of occasions) a conduction defect unless there is an air–bone gap of at least 30 dB and more probably 40 dB.

An alternative and more encouraging way to look at the data is that if the bone conduction is louder than the air conduction then there is likely to be an air–bone gap of 10 dB or more. This is different from saying that the Rinne test will detect a conductive defect, as it is only when the air–bone gap is greater than 40 dB that it will be detected on 90 per cent of occasions. The reason why practising otologists have come to believe that the Rinne test is more reliable than this is that when the bone conduction is louder than the air conduction (Rinne negative) there is usually an air–bone gap. The above figures support this but what the otologist tends to forget is the considerable number of occasions when there is an air–bone gap and a Rinne negative response is not obtained.

Clinical role

What the otologist needs to know in a patient with a hearing impairment is whether there is

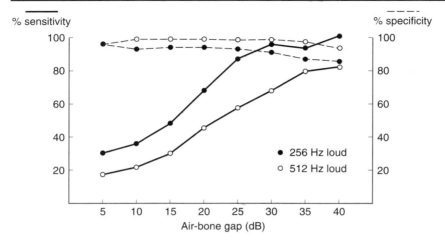

Figure 2.5 Sensitivity and specificity of 256 Hz (●) and 512 Hz (O) tuning forks in detecting differences in air and bone conduction of various magnitudes (after Browning *et al.*, 1989)

Table 2.6 Size of air–bone gap (dB) which would be correctly identified by Rinne test on various percentages of occasions

| | *Confidence limits* | | |
	50%	*75%*	*90+%*
256 Hz fork:			
Crowley and Kaufman (1966)	25		30
Gelfand (1977)		40	
512 Hz fork:			
Crowley and Kaufman (1966)	25		30
Wilson and Woods (1975)			40
Gelfand (1977)		40	
Golabek and Stephens (1979)	19		
Browning and Swan (1988)	20		45

a conductive component and, if this is the case, what is its magnitude. The latter question can only be determined by pure tone audiometry with masking. The Rinne test does not help to determine the magnitude of an air–bone gap, it is only an aid to determining whether there is a conduction defect. In patients with otoscopic evidence of middle ear pathology, such as chronic otitis media, by definition there must be a conduction defect and the Rinne test adds nothing. However, when the tympanic membrane is normal and the bone conduction is louder than the air conduction (Rinne negative) there is most likely a conduction defect. In adults this would suggest otosclerosis. If the air conduction is louder than bone conduction (Rinne positive) in these circumstances there could still be a conductive defect due to otosclerosis of a magnitude that could benefit from surgery.

Weber test

Why this test is so popular is uncertain as it can only really be interpreted when there is a unilateral hearing impairment. One of the main problems with this test is that the response is not reproducible, as can be verified by retesting a patient. Different results are frequently obtained if the base of the fork is positioned on the nasion or on the upper lip rather than on the vertex.

Most publications would agree that the results of the Weber test are difficult to interpret when there is a bilateral hearing impairment. So, assuming that it is known that a patient has a unilateral hearing impairment, how accurate is the Weber test in deciding whether it is a sensorineural or a conductive impairment? In 30 per cent of cases the test will be referred to the mid-line so the result cannot be interpreted as being correct or incorrect. Of the 70 per cent who do refer the test to one ear, about 25 per cent refer it to the incorrect ear (Stankiewicz and Mowry, 1979). It is concluded that the Weber test is likely to add little to the assessment in the majority of patients.

Other tuning fork tests

Many other tests have been described and are well summarized by Hinchcliffe (1981) but are infrequently used.

This is mainly because they were developed before audiometric testing was possible. Now that accurate audiometry is almost universally available, they are of historical interest only. The Weber test in the author's opinion comes in the same category.

■ Conclusions

• Clinical assessment of a patient's hearing by free-field speech can be helpful in many ways. It is wise to have the severity of an impairment clinically assessed as audiometry can on occasions be inaccurate or not available. In many instances the degree of accuracy that audiometry gives may be unnecessary, for example, in screening the elderly for hearing aid provision. Exaggerated thresholds may be missed if suspicion is not aroused by clinical testing. In addition, it considerably aids the interpretation of tuning fork tests if these are carried out.
• Masking is as important in clinical testing as it is in audiometric testing.
• Tragal rubbing is the easiest and most appropriate method of masking to use routinely as it requires no instruments and there is no risk of overmasking.
• A Barany box can potentially overmask the test ear. In free-field voice testing it should only be used when there is a unilateral profound loss of hearing and in tuning fork testing when a bilateral conductive impairment is likely.
• If a patient can hear a whispered voice at a distance of 2 feet, his pure tone average (PTA) threshold is likely to be better than 30 dB HL.
• Free-field speech testing can divide the severity of a hearing impairment into three bands: normal; mild/moderate; severe/profound. This is sufficiently accurate for many purposes.
• The Rinne test is less reliable in detecting a conductive defect than we would like to believe. Though the cross-over point from Rinne positive to negative is an air–bone gap of ~ 20 dB, this means that 50 per cent of individuals with a gap of this size will be Rinne positive (air conduction louder than bone conduction).
• The Rinne test will not reliably detect (90 per cent confidence) an air–bone gap until it is 40 dB or greater.
• On the other hand, if the bone conduction is louder than the air conduction (Rinne negative) there will be an air–bone gap of 10 dB or greater. However, a considerable proportion of ears with clinically important air–bone gaps will not give this result.
• The Weber test is only interpretable when

there is a unilateral impairment and, because of its error rate of 25 per cent when it is referred to one ear, it is considered to add little to the clinical assessment.

- In the detection and quantification of a conductive defect reliance will have to be primarily on pure tone audiometry rather than on tuning fork tests.

Further reading

Browning, G.G. (1987). Guest Editorial. Is there still a role for tuning-fork tests? *British Journal of Audiology*, **21**, 161–163.

Swan, I.R.C. (1997). Clinical tests of hearing and balance. In *Adult Audiology*, Vol. 2, Chap. 5, Scott-Brown's Otolaryngology, 6th Edition. Butterworth-Heinemann, Oxford.

Wormald, P.J. and Browning, G.G. (1996). *Otoscopy – A Structured Approach*. Arnold, London.

3 Pure tone audiometry

Aims

Pure tone audiometry is the basic audiometric test which assesses the thresholds for air and bone conduction over a range of pure tones for each ear. These thresholds are usually charted on an audiogram and can be used: (a) to assess the degree of impairment in each ear; and, if one is present, (b) to ascertain whether it is conductive, sensorineural or mixed in type.

Audiogram

The standard pure tone audiogram chart (*Figure 3.1*) has the test frequencies on the horizontal axis and the thresholds of hearing on the vertical axis. The standard test frequencies are at octave intervals from 0.25 to 8 kHz (250–8000 Hz). Testing can also be done at other frequencies, but 3 and 6 kHz are the commonest additional frequencies, particularly in the assessment of sensorineural impairments. The vertical axis is in decibels hearing level (dB HL) with a range from −10 to 120 dB HL, the latter being the greatest sound level that can be generated by most audiometers over headphones. Some audiometers, particularly portable ones, are less powerful. The dB HL scale was designed so that 0 dB HL at each frequency, for air and bone conduction, represented the mean thresholds of 'normal' hearing. This was done to make interpretation easier, as the auditory system is less efficient at detecting sounds at some frequencies. *Figure 3.2* shows the level of detection of sounds in decibels of sound pressure level (dB SPL) of the human ear. In this decibel scale there is an equal amount of energy (in dynes/cm^2) at each frequency. Because of the U-shaped nature of this audiogram, it was considered that the use of a dB SPL scale in an audiogram would make abnormalities difficult to identify. Hence, it was decided to create a biological scale of human hearing so that 0 dB HL would be the expected threshold of detection of a pure tone irrespective of its frequency. The amount of energy at 0 dB HL at each frequency is not the same, the levels being initially achieved by testing otologically normal, young

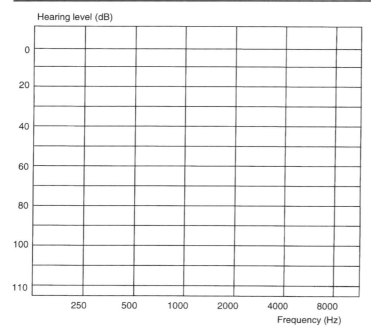

Figure 3.1 Standard audiogram chart

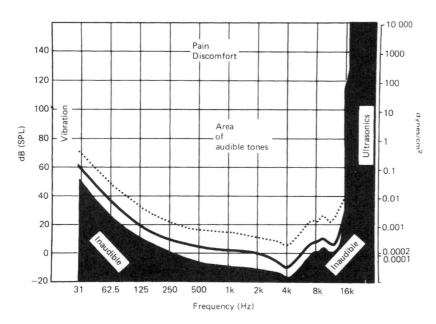

Figure 3.2 Normal sound pressure levels of detection of pure tones in humans. Solid line = median levels; broken line = upper 90th percentile (after Robinson and Dadson, 1957)

adults. Unfortunately 'normal' was not the same in every country and different standards in relation to dB SPL were created. These differences were resolved by the International Standards Organisation in 1964 (ISO, 1964) and their standards are now universally used. So in the dB HL scale normal hearing individuals would be expected to have a flat audiogram, the mean level being 0 dB HL.

In industrial situations, portable instruments are used to measure noise, but they, like the ear, do not measure as efficiently at some frequencies as others. Over the years several weighted dB noise scales have been used for these instruments but the current one is dB A.

Recommended manual technique

There are many different ways of manually assessing the air- and bone-conduction thresholds but the British Society of Audiology's recommended procedures (Appendix II) would be acceptable in most departments, both in and outside the UK. Many aspects require some comment.

Test environment

Without spending a considerable amount of money it is impossible to exclude all extraneous sound from the test environment. The sound level in a 'quiet' room is seldom less than 30 dB A and often 40–50 dB A. Background noise acts as a masking noise and can appreciably influence the results in normal individuals, especially bone conduction at low frequencies. The commonest cause of a low frequency hearing loss is thus insufficient exclusion of background noise from the test environment in a normal individual (*Figure 3.3*). Background noise can be lessened by several means:

- sound attenuating headphones;
- sound deadening of the test room;
- use of an acoustic booth.

Calibration

The sound level output of both the air- and bone-conduction modes of an audiometer can change with time which means that an audiometer needs to be calibrated and adjusted regularly, preferably every 6 months.

Threshold determination

The term threshold means the minimum level at which a signal can be detected. However, these can differ depending on the techniques being used to determine them. Firstly, the thresholds obtained will depend on whether they are assessed by ascending from the inaudible until they become audible or descending from the audible until they become inaudible. The recommended procedure is a tracking one, ascending and descending about the threshold until positive responses have been made on 50 per cent or more of the occasions the signal has been presented at a specific dB HL. Secondly, it is important to instruct the patient to respond 'at the least suggestion of a signal' rather than 'when the signal is definitely heard'. If the patient responds in the second manner the threshold can be 5–15 dB higher.

Reproducibility

In testing air conduction at any one frequency, the test/retest variation is no greater than ± 5 dB, so taken as an average over four frequencies, any change in the pure tone average of 5 dB or greater between two test occasions is significant, provided the machine has been calibrated and the test environment is similar. In testing bone conduction, because of the additional variables such as positioning and pressure of the vibrator, the test/retest variation can be much greater. Mean changes of bone conduction of 10–15 dB on different test occasions have to be interpreted with caution.

Because 0 dB HL by definition indicates normal hearing in young adults, the air-conduction and bone-conduction thresholds should be the same in normal hearing individuals (they are not the same in tuning fork tests). This is also the case in those with a sensorineural impairment where the sound-conduction mechanism of the external and middle ears is normal. In those with a conductive impairment, the bone-conduction thresholds will be better than the air-conduction thresholds, the magnitude of

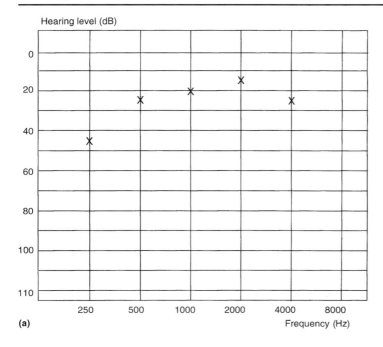

(a)

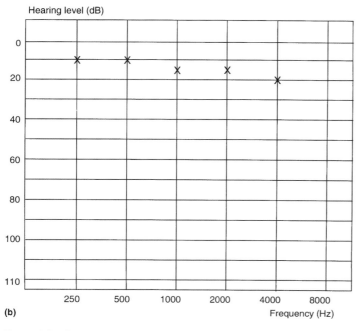

(b)

Figure 3.3 Effect of noisy test situations on hearing in normal individuals. (a) Upper 95th percentile of hearing in a group of patients tested in a noisy casualty ward; (b) upper 95th percentile of hearing in these same patients when tested in an acoustic booth

the difference being the air–bone gap. Because of test/retest error, air–bone gaps of 10 dB or less are not considered significant and are usually disregarded.

Test order

The air-conduction thresholds in the better hearing ear (if any) are tested first, usually starting at 1 kHz, and then at 2, 4, 8, 0.25 and 0.5 kHz. The air-conduction thresholds are then assessed in the other ear in the same order. The right air-conduction thresholds are indicated by an O and the left by an X. Coloured pens are sometimes used, with red representing right and blue representing left. To ease interpretation, in some departments the thresholds for each ear are recorded on separate charts. If the air-conduction thresholds are 40 dB or more different between ears, it is then necessary to mask the better hearing ear and retest the poorer ear in case the thresholds in that ear are a mirror of the better ear (see below).

The not-masked bone-conduction thresholds are then recorded at 1 and then 2, 4, 0.5 and 0.25 kHz with the vibrator on the side of the better air-conduction thresholds, if any. The reason for choosing this side is that the not-masked bone conduction thresholds are most likely to apply to that ear, the not-masked bone-conduction thresholds being the best bone-conduction thresholds in any patient. The reason that bone conduction is not tested at 8 kHz is that the output is insufficient at this frequency. Following this, the audiogram can be classified into one of three groups to decide whether it is necessary to mask the bone conduction: no potential air–bone gap, potential air–bone gap, definite air–bone gap.

No potential air–bone gap

If the air-conduction thresholds in both ears and the not-masked bone-conduction thresholds are within 10 dB of each other at all frequencies, there is no potential air–bone gap in either ear. This occurs in individuals with normal hearing (*Figure 3.4*) or in those with a bilateral, symmetric sensorineural impairment (*Figure 3.5*). There is no need to go on to assess the bone-conduction thresholds separately in each ear. No other result is possible as the not-masked bone-conduction thresh-

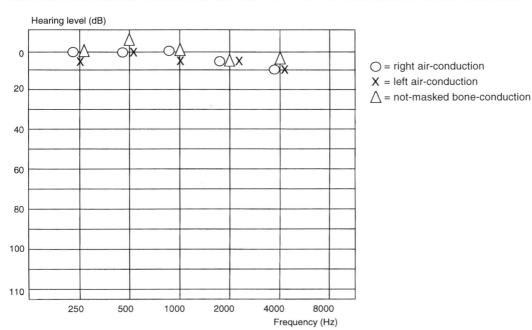

O = right air-conduction
X = left air-conduction
△ = not-masked bone-conduction

Figure 3.4 Normal hearing in both ears, that is the air-conduction thresholds are less than 25 dB HL. The not-masked bone-conduction thresholds are less than 10 dB different from any of the air-conduction thresholds. There is thus no potential air–bone gap and no need to mask the bone conduction

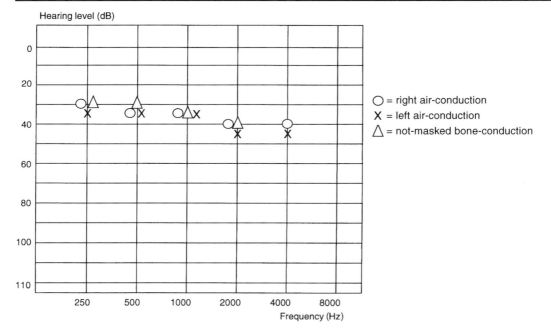

Figure 3.5 Bilateral, symmetrical sensorineural impairment. The pure tone average in the right ear is $35 + 35 + 40 + 50 = 160 \div 4 = 40$ dB HL and in the left ear is $35 + 35 + 45 + 50 = 165 \div 4 = 41$ dB HL. That is, both ears have a mild impairment. At all frequencies the not-masked bone-conduction thresholds are less than 10 dB different from the air-conduction thresholds in either ear. There is thus no potential air–bone gap in either ear and no need to mask the bone-conduction

olds are the best possible thresholds achievable in any patient.

Definite air–bone gap

Where the not-masked bone-conduction thresholds are better than the air-conduction thresholds by 10 dB or more in *both* ears, then there must be an air–bone gap in one or both ears (*Figure 3.6*). This is because the not-masked bone-conduction thresholds apply to at least one ear, so by definition an air–bone gap must exist in at least one ear. Masking is required to assess the bone-conduction thresholds in each ear.

Potential air–bone gap

When the not-masked bone-conduction thresholds are the same as the air-conduction thresholds in one ear but not the other (*Figure 3.7*) the not-masked bone-conduction thresholds must apply to the better ear. Potentially there could be an air–bone gap or a sensorineural impairment in the poorer ear, so masking of the better ear is required to assess the bone-conduction thresholds in the poorer ear.

Bone-conduction masking

The bone-conduction vibrator vibrates the entire skull and, hence, both cochleas. It is agreed that, regardless of where the bone vibrator is placed, there is no way of knowing which ear is being tested unless masking is used. Some (Stevens, 1981) suggest that the not-masked bone-conduction thresholds be assessed with the vibrator on the vertex to remind the tester of this but in many instances this can lead to considerably higher thresholds. *Table 3.1* shows the transcranial attenua-

Table 3.1 Transcranial attenuation (dB)

Bone conduction	Mean	0.5 kHz	1 kHz	2 kHz	4 kHz
Minimum	−6	−10	−5	−5	−5
Maximum	31	25	25	35	40
Median	10	10	5	10	15

(After Snyder, 1973)

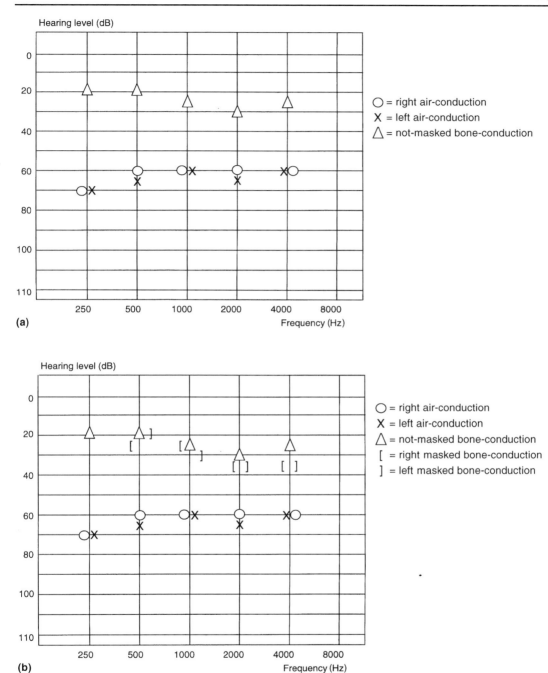

Figure 3.6 (a) Potential air–bone gap in one or both ears. This patient has a bilateral moderate impairment, the pure tone average in the right ear being 60 dB HL and in the left ear 63 dB HL. The not-masked bone-conduction thresholds are in the region of 25 dB HL and could apply to either or both ears. Masking is required to ascertain the masked bone-conduction thresholds. The most likely outcome is that there is a bilateral conductive impairment (b). A much less likely alternative is that there is a conductive impairment in one ear and a sensorineural (or mixed) impairment in the other ear of the same magnitude (c)

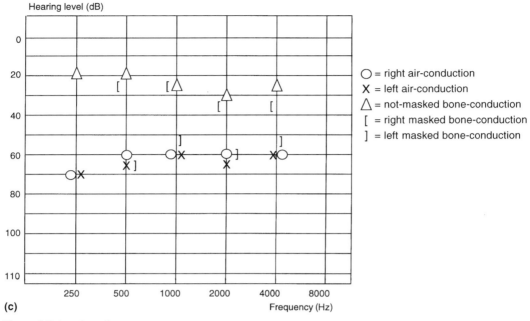

(c)

Figure 3.6 (*continued*)

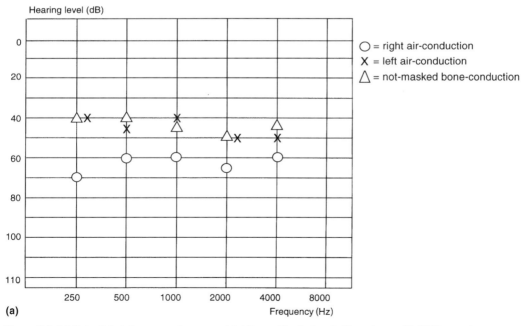

(a)

Figure 3.7 (a) Potential air-bone gap in poorer (right) ear. The better (left) ear has a 46 dB HL pure tone average and the not-masked bone-conduction thresholds at all frequencies are less than 10 dB different from the air-conduction thresholds and these must apply to the left ear. The right ear has a 61 dB HL average and the left ear air-conduction has to be masked so that the masked bone-conduction thresholds can be assessed. The two most likely outcomes are that there is a mixed loss in the right ear (b) or a sensorineural loss in the right ear (c)

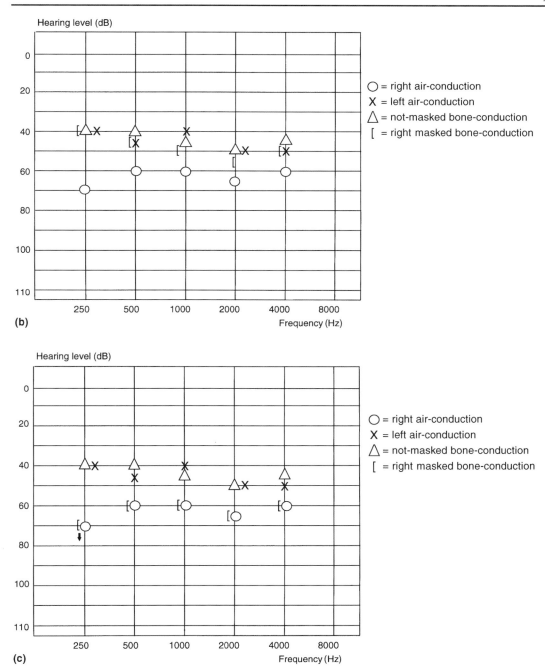

Figure 3.7 (*continued*)

tion of bone conduction from one side of the skull to the other. The range of values is quite large and indeed can be better for the ear on the opposite side to the one being stimulated. As it is not possible to predict what the value will be in an individual patient, the minimum values have to be assumed. These are less than 0 dB at every frequency. Hence, whenever one desires to assess the bone conduction in an ear with a potential air–bone gap, it is necessary to mask the bone conduction in the other ear. This cannot be done by bone conduction as this will mask the bone conduction in the test ear as well. Hence it has to be done by air, usually with an ear insert rather than headphones.

Several different methods of masking have been proposed but the preferred method is shadow masking and to record the thresholds on a masking chart (*Figure 3.8*). The masking signal is a narrow band of noise in the region of the test frequency. It is usual to start with the masking sound at its threshold of detection in the non-test ear. If the threshold in the test ear deteriorates with this level of masking, cross-hearing is occurring and the level of masking is increased by 10 dB and the threshold re-assessed. This procedure is repeated until the thresholds are no longer affected by an increase in masking level. The true threshold is the level where three sequential masking levels give rise to thresholds that are within 5 dB (*Figure 3.8*). If the masking sound is increased any further, the thresholds will start to deteriorate, initially because of central masking and then because of cross-masking. The reason why the central masking occurs is uncertain but its contribution is unimportant in practice compared with cross-masking when the masking sound is sufficiently loud that it masks the test ear as well.

Air-conduction masking

Having carried out any bone-conduction masking to confirm whether an air–bone gap is present or not, it is now necessary to reconsider whether any air-conduction masking is required. This may already have been considered necessary and have been carried out after the air-conduction thresholds had been determined and a difference of 40 dB or greater noted.

To understand air-conduction masking it is necessary to realize that the tones are presented via headphones and not free-field. The amount of sound that escapes from these headphones is negligible but what they do is vibrate the skull. Sound can then go by bone conduction from the headphone on one side to the cochlea on the other side. Inevitably because of the mass of the skull the sound will be attenuated to a certain degree and for practical purposes the minimum level is taken as 40 dB (*Figure 3.9*). There are two main situations when this might affect the air-conduction thresholds.

(1) If there is a difference of more than 40 dB between the air conduction in the poorer ear and the bone-conduction (which is often also the same as the air conduction) in the better ear, the air-conduction thresholds in the poorer ear could be a shadow from the better ear (see *Figures 3.10* and *3.11*). Repeat air-conduction testing,

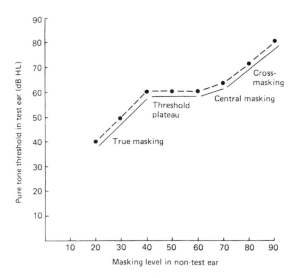

Figure 3.8 Masking chart

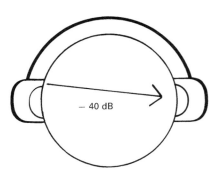

Figure 3.9 Trans-skull attenuation of headphone air-conduction sounds. The sound arrives at the cochlea on the non-test side attenuated by 40 dB or greater

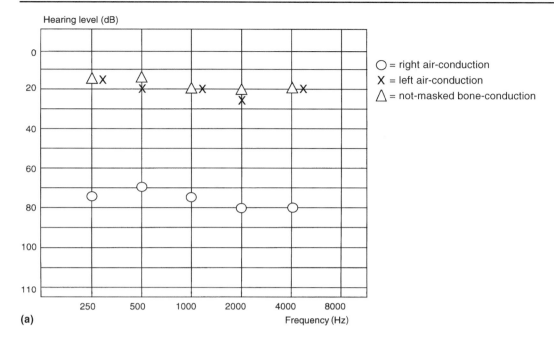

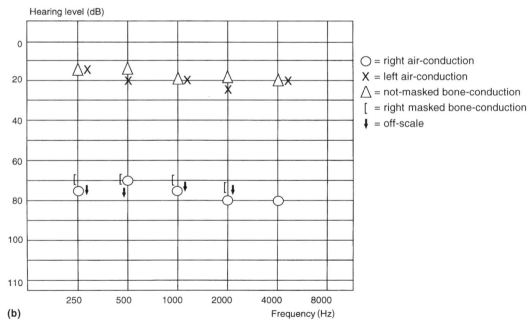

Figure 3.10 (a) Requirement to mask the air conduction. The pure tone average in the left ear is 21 dB HL, which is normal. At all frequencies the not-masked bone-conduction thresholds are less than 10 dB different from the air-conduction thresholds and hence these must apply to the left ear. The pure tone average in the right ear is 76 dB HL. These thresholds could be a shadow from the left ear and the first requirement is to mask the air conduction in the left ear and assess the masked bone-conduction thresholds in the right ear. In this instance they are off-scale (b). It is still possible that the right air-conduction thresholds might be due to transcranial hearing in the left ear because the air-conduction thresholds in the poorer ear are more than 40 dB worse than the bone conduction in the better ear. In this instance when the air conduction in the right ear is reassessed the right ear is a 'dead' ear (c)

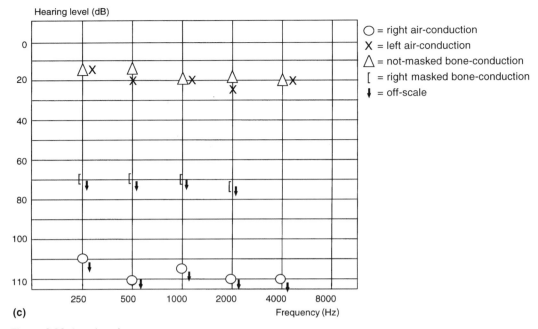

(c)

Figure 3.10 (*continued*)

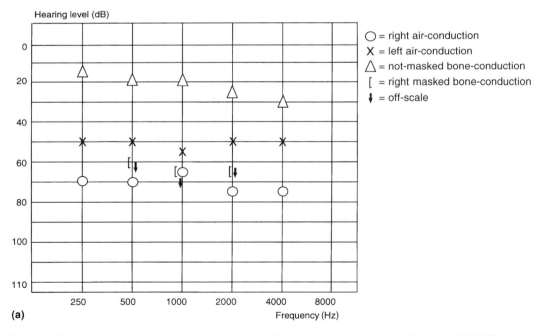

(a)

Figure 3.11 (a) Requirement to mask the air-conduction. The pure tone average in the left ear is 51 dB HL and in the right is 71 dB HL. The not-masked bone-conduction thresholds are likely to apply to the left ear and masking confirms this in that the masked bone-conduction thresholds in the right ear are off-scale. There is now a requirement to mask the left ear and assess the masked air-conduction thresholds because the air-conduction thresholds in the poorer (right) ear are worse than the bone conduction in the better (left) ear by greater than 40 dB. Having done this, the patient is found to have a profound rather than a severe sensorineural impairment in the right ear (b)

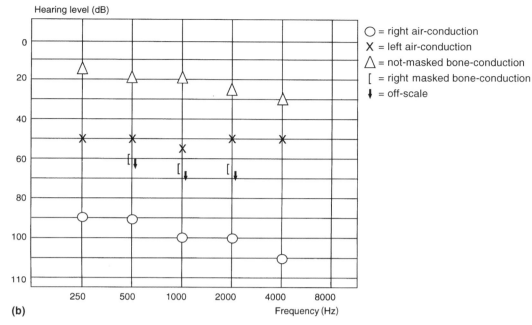

(b)

Figure 3.11 (*continued*)

with masking of the better ear, will be necessary.

(2) If there is a major conductive defect in the test ear, the air-conduction thresholds could be the threshold of detection of the sound from the headphones via the osseous route (*Figure 3.11*). In these circumstances the air–bone gap would not necessarily be an accurate measure of the magnitude of the conductive defect.

Air-conduction masking is again a narrow-band noise in the region of the test frequency but delivered by headphones. The same shadow masking procedure is used as in bone-conduction masking.

Interpreting the audiogram

Pure tone average (PTA)

The first assessment is of the air-conduction thresholds in each ear which is usually done by averaging the thresholds over 0.5, 1, 2 and 4 kHz to give a four frequency PTA. For some purposes a three frequency average over 1, 2 and 3 kHz is used (see p. 52). It is then possible to categorize the degree of hearing impairment in each ear using one of the recognized bandings (*Table 3.2*).

A decision is also made as to whether the thresholds are symmetric (within 10 dB of each other) or asymmetric (different by greater than 10 dB). This distinction does not always agree with a patient's report as to how symmetric the hearing is. There are many potential reasons for this but a stricter pure tone threshold criterion cannot be used because of the 10 dB test/retest error of audiometry.

In most patients, the PTA is not formally calculated, as the degree of impairment can usually be assessed by 'eyeballing' the audiogram. Calculating the PTA is often left for

Table 3.2 Classification used to describe the degree of hearing impairment

Degree of impairment	Hearing* (dB HL)
None	< 26
Mild	26–40
Moderate	41–55
Moderately severe	56–70
Severe	71–90
Profound	91–110
Total	> 110

*'Hearing' is the mean of the thresholds over 0.5, 1, 2 and 4 kHz

specific circumstances, such as when a report is being written, for research and when the PTA is borderline between categories of impairments.

Type of impairment

There are four types of impairment that can be identified audiometrically: conductive, sensorineural, mixed and uncertain.

Conductive impairment

This is considered present if there is an air–bone gap of greater than 10 dB, usually averaged over 0.5, 1 and 2 kHz rather than 0.5, 1, 2 and 4 kHz (*Figure 3.12*). In most cases the air–bone gap is greatest at the lower frequencies for the reasons explained in Chapter 3. An ear with an air–bone gap of less than 10 dB does not necessarily have a normal conductive mechanism, it is just that an impairment cannot be measured because of the test/retest error of the method (*Figure 3.13*).

Sensorineural impairment

Here there is no air–bone gap, but the PTA is worse than the level considered to be 'normal'. What defines 'normal' is debated. Criteria can be set which, if satisfied, categorize the patient as having normal hearing. Such a criterion is a pure tone average over 0.5, 1, 2 and 4 kHz of 25 or 30 dB HL (*Figure 3.4*). Criteria can also be set which, if the thresholds fail, categorize the patient as having abnormal hearing. Such a criterion is that there is an

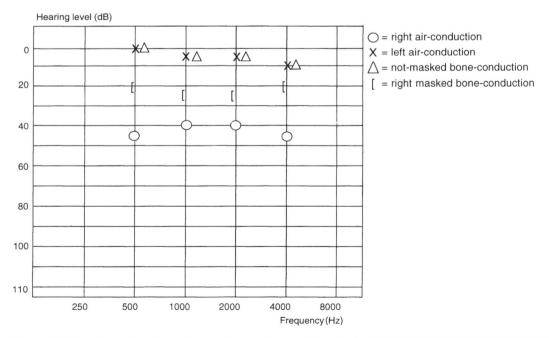

Figure 3.12 Conductive impairment in the right ear with normal hearing in the left ear. The not-masked bone-conduction thresholds must apply to the left ear. Masking of the air conduction in the left ear is necessary to assess the masked bone-conduction thresholds in the right ear. The pure tone average in the right ear is 45 + 40 + 40 + 45 = 170 ÷ 4 = 43 dB HL. The air–bone gap in the right ear is 25 + 15 + 15 = 55 ÷ 3 = 18 dB HL

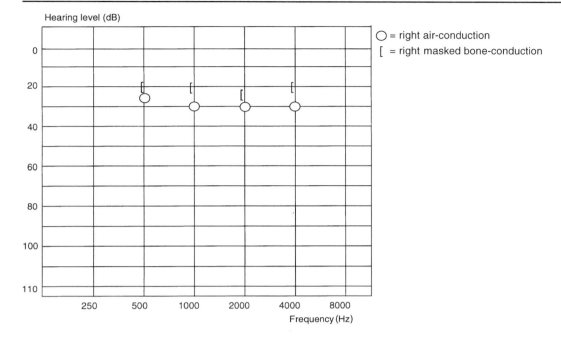

Figure 3.13 Unlikely conductive impairment. The air–bone gap is $5 + 10 + 5 = 20 \div 3 = 7$ dB HL

impairment if the threshold at any single frequency is poorer than a certain level, often taken again as 25 or 30 dB HL (*Figure 3.5*). Sensorineural impairments usually affect the high frequencies rather than the low ones, giving rise to a sloping audiogram (*Figure 3.14*). Sometimes there is a notch in the audiogram around 4 kHz (*Figure 3.5*) but this may not be identified unless 3 and 6 kHz are tested as well (*Figure 3.15*). The presence of a notch is not unusual in ears with a mild to moderate sensorineural hearing impairment. This can occur whatever the aetiology, though some would suggest that it is more likely as a consequence of noise trauma.

Mixed impairment

Here there is both a conductive and a sensori-neural impairment in an ear. The criterion for a conductive component is again an air–bone gap of greater than 10 dB and for a sensorineural component an average bone-conduction threshold worse than a certain 'normal' criterion, usually 25 or 30 dB HL. The level of bone-conduction thresholds used to define 'normal' in a mixed impairment is even

more debated than with a sensorineural impairment because of the Carhart effect (see below). It could be argued that the level should be poorer than the 25–30 dB HL pure-tone average usually taken. However, in most instances no allowance is made for the Carhart effect.

Uncertain type

In patients with a severe or profound impairment, it is not unusual to be uncertain as to whether the impairment is sensorineural or mixed in type. This is for two reasons that apply only to this group. First, the maximum bone-conduction output of most audiometers is in the region of 70 dB. It can be even less in portable audiometers. Hence, if the not-masked bone-conduction thresholds are poorer than this, they cannot be assessed (*Figure 3.10b* and *c*). All ears with a profound impairment (PTA ⩾ 90 dB HL) could therefore have either a sensorineural or mixed impairment if the bone-conduction thresholds are poorer than 70 dB HL (*Figure 3.16*). Secondly, the maximum output available to mask bone conduction is usually 110 dB. This greatly limits

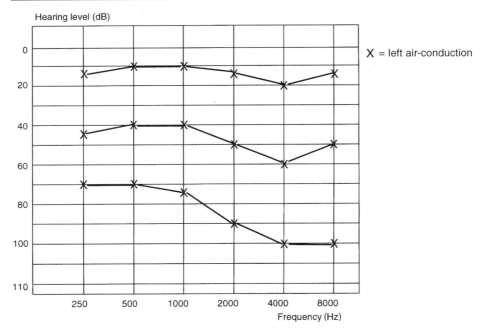

Figure 3.14 Typical progression of a sensorineural impairment. This example shows three sequential air-conduction audiograms in the left ear. Bone-conduction thresholds are omitted for simplicity

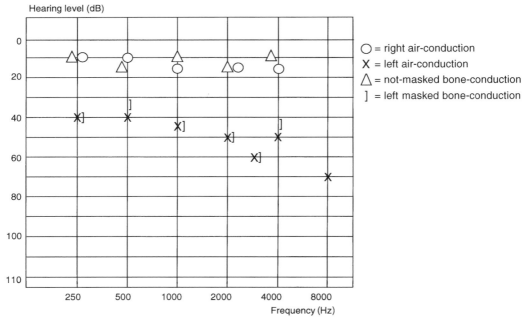

Figure 3.15 Notch in audiogram at 3 kHz in the left ear which has a mild sensorineural hearing impairment. This would not have been evident if the thresholds at 3 kHz had not been tested

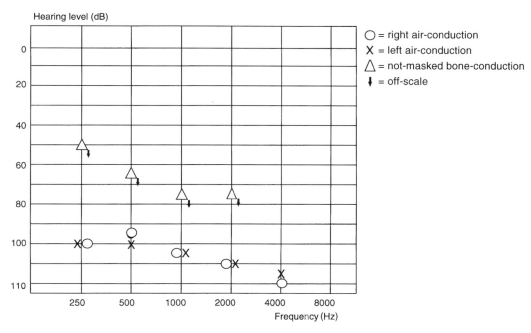

Figure 3.16 Bilateral profound impairment where it is not possible to ascertain the type of impairment because of limited output of bone-conduction. It could be a mixed or a pure sensorineural impairment

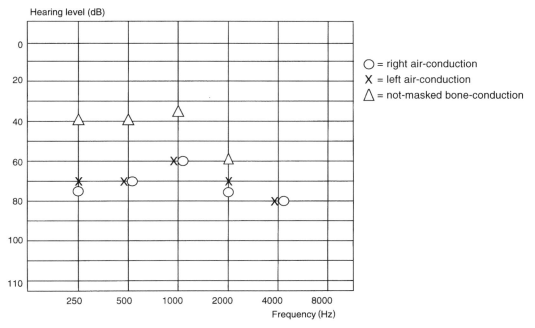

Figure 3.17 Bilateral severe impairment. One or both ears have a mixed impairment but it is uncertain which because of an inability to mask due to the limited output of masking noise; that is, 110 dB is insufficient to mask the hearing in an ear with a pure tone average of 70 dB HL

the amount of masking available when the air-conduction thresholds are poorer than 70 dB HL (*Figure 3.16*). Thus in patients with a bilateral severe (or poorer) impairment in whom some not-masked bone-conduction thresholds are available, it is not possible to get masked bone-conduction thresholds to decide whether both or only one ear has a conductive component (*Figure 3.17*). Further examples are considered in *Figures 11.1–11.5*.

Inner ear function

Often an assessment of inner ear function or 'cochlear reserve' is required. The most fre-

quent reason is in compensation claims for noise-induced deafness where the object is to compare a claimant's sensorineural thresholds with those of 'normal' controls, matched for age, sex and socio-economic group. The other reason is to assess the potential benefit from middle ear surgery to improve the hearing if the air–bone gap is closed.

In patients with no air–bone gap, the air-conduction thresholds are taken to represent inner ear function and this is valid. In those with an air–bone gap, this is not the case and the only alternative is to use the bone-conduction thresholds. However, when there is a conduction defect, the bone-conduction thresholds do not assess the same things as they normally would.

What are the bone-conduction thresholds?

Hearing by bone conduction helps one to monitor one's own voice. Its assessment in audiometry is of value in detecting and quantifying conduction defects, but when such a defect is present the bone-conduction thresholds underestimate inner ear function.

When the skull is set in vibration by bone-conducted sounds this reaches the inner ear by three routes (*Figure 3.18*). Firstly, the sound emanates into the external auditory canal and is

heard via the middle ear (route c). Secondly, the skull vibration sets the ossicular chain in motion and this energy is transferred to the inner ear via the middle ear (route b). Thirdly, the cochlea vibrates along with the skull and this stimulates the inner ear (route a). It is difficult to ascertain the relative contribution of each of those routes, but those going via the external auditory canal and middle ear are likely to be as important as the direct one (*Figure 3.19*).

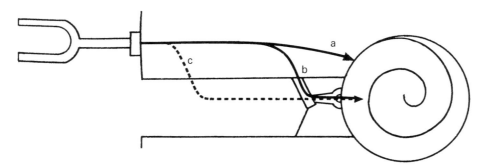

Figure 3.18 The three routes of bone conduction to the cochlea: (a) via skull vibration; (b) via ossicular chain vibration; (c) via the external auditory canal

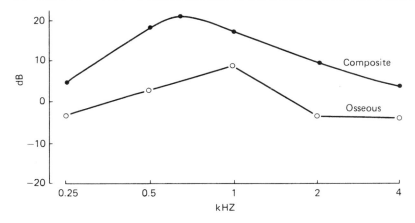

Figure 3.19 The composite cochlear microphonics at various frequencies in cats initiated by stimulating bone conduction. The osseous component is that which arrives at the inner ear via the bone. The remainder is made up of the components arriving at the inner ear via the external auditory canal and the middle ear (after Tonndorf, 1972)

In ears with a conductive defect, the sound will not be as well transmitted by the first two routes, leading to poorer bone-conduction thresholds in such ears. This Carhart effect, which is more fully discussed in Chapter 4, p. 43, occurs at all frequencies but is maximal at 2 kHz. The implication is that in an ear with a conductive impairment the bone-conduction thresholds are not a measure of inner ear function in the same way that they are in a normal ear or one with a sensorineural impairment.

■ Conclusions

- Pure tone audiometry is the standard audiometric test.
- If carried out in a sound deadened environment, with calibrated equipment, using a standard technique in a patient who responds when they 'think they can hear a tone', the results are highly reproducible.
- The results can be used to define in each ear the air-conduction thresholds for pure tones. When averaged these give an indication of the degree of impairment in each ear.
- If the bone-conduction thresholds are better than the air-conduction thresholds, as evidenced by an air–bone gap of 10 dB or greater, there is a defect in the sound-conduction mechanism of the external and/or middle ear.
- Bone-conduction thresholds are initially assessed not-masked. When there is a potential air–bone gap in an ear, the bone-conduction thresholds need to be reassessed with masking of the other ear.
- A sensorineural hearing impairment is considered to be present if the bone-conduction thresholds are similar to the air-conduction thresholds and the average of the latter (usually over 0.5, 1, 2 and 4 kHz) is worse than a certain level which defines normal hearing, usually 25 or 30 dB HL.
- A mixed hearing impairment is considered to be present if the average bone-conduction thresholds satisfy the definition for a sensorineural impairment and there is in addition an air–bone gap of 10 dB or greater.
- When the air-conduction thresholds in the poorer hearing ear are worse than the bone-conduction thresholds in the contralateral ear by 40 dB or more, the air-conduction thresholds could be a shadow of these bone-conduction thresholds and must be masked.
- The bone-conduction thresholds do not

measure solely inner ear function. In a normal ear and in those with a sensorineural impairment, there is also a material air-conduction component transmitted via the external canal and ossicular chain.

• In those with a conductive impairment, the bone-conduction thresholds do not have this air-conduction component. This Carhart effect occurs at all frequencies but is greatest at 2 kHz.

Further reading

British Society of Audiology (1981). Recommended procedures for pure-tone audiometry using a manually operated instrument. *British Journal of Audiology*, **15**, 213–216.

British Society of Audiology (1985). Technical note: Recommended procedure for pure tone bone-conduction audiometry without masking using a manually operated instrument. *British Journal of Audiology*, **19**, 281–282.

British Society of Audiology (1986). Technical note: Recommendations for masking in pure tone threshold audiometry. *British Journal of Audiology*, **20**, 307–314.

4 Conductive defects

Identification of pathology

The otologist, when he sees a patient with a hearing impairment, will diagnose the majority of pathologies in the external auditory canal and middle ear by otoscopy, the main exception being otosclerosis. On some occasions the tympanic membrane may be difficult to assess and tympanometry can be of value. In those with evident canal or middle ear pathology, the air–bone gap in pure-tone audiometry will quantify the magnitude of the conductive impairment. The degree of impairment will be assessed from the air-conduction (a-c) thresholds. Sometimes, when otoscopy is normal, the audiogram will suggest a conductive impairment. The task then is to confirm that this is indeed the case and to reach a diagnosis.

Prevalence of middle ear pathology

The British MRC National Study of Hearing assessed the prevalence, in adults over the age of 18 years, of middle ear disease in the early 1980s (*Table 4.1*). Otoscopically 12 per cent (95 per cent confidence interval) (CI 10.2–13.6) had healed otitis media, 2.6 per cent (CI 1.8–3.4) had inactive chronic otitis

Table 4.1 Prevalence in adult population (per cent) of chronic otitis media and otosclerosis (the 95 per cent confidence limits are given in parentheses)

| | Chronic otitis media | | Otosclerosis |
	Active	*Inactive*	
Overall prevalence	2.5 (2–3.5)	1.5 (1–2)	2 (1.5–3)
Age grouping:			
18–40 years	2.5 (1–4)	1 (0.5–1.5)	1.5 (1–3)
41–60 years	2 (1–3)	2 (1–3)	2 (1–3)
61–80 years	3 (2–4)	2 (1–3)	3 (1–4)
Sex grouping:			
Women	2.5 (2–3)	1 (0.5–1.5)	2 (1–3)
Men	3 (1.5–4)	2 (1–3)	2 (1–3)
Occupational grouping:			
Non-manual	2 (1–3)	1 (0–1)	1.5 (1–2)
Manual	3 (2–4)	2 (1.5–3)	3 (2–4)

(After Browning and Gatehouse, 1992)

media and 1.5 per cent (CI 1.1–1.9) had active chronic otitis media. Unfortunately the patients with active chronic otitis media could not be broken down into cholesteatoma and mucosal disease. Defining otosclerosis as a normal tympanic membrane and normal middle ear pressure, but with an air–bone gap of 15 dB over 0.5, 1 and 2 kHz, 2 per cent (CI 1.5–2.7) of the population had the condition.

Wax (cerumen)

The otoscopist has to be aware that what sometimes appears to be wax is not wax at all. Dried pus and squamous debris are frequently brown and can be confused with wax, particularly in mastoid cavities.

The inexperienced frequently consider wax to be the cause of a conductive impairment. Wax is secreted by the ceruminous glands in the cartilagenous, outer one-third of the canal. Normally, wax is shed along with dead squamous epithelium from the skin of the canal by migration of the epithelium. Sound vibrations are not usually impeded in the canal unless it is so occluded that the vibrations cannot pass through. Ear plugs worn for sound protection work in this manner, provided they are pressed right in. Wax in the outer third of the canal is never sufficiently occlusive to achieve this effect. However, if impacted by a finger, cotton bud or mould of a hearing aid deep in the canal, it may do so (*Figure 4.1*). Impacted wax against the tympanic membrane may sometimes also directly inhibit movement. Debris on the tympanic membrane may affect its loading and its frequency response but seldom

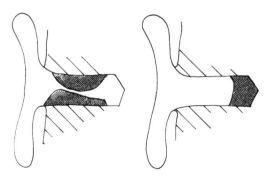

Figure 4.1 The wax on the left would not cause an acoustic obstruction, whereas that on the right would

causes a hearing impairment. This is in contra-distinction to a drop of water, which will immobilize it by surface tension, in the same way as middle ear fluid does in otitis media with effusion.

Otitis externa

Otitis externa seldom causes a significant impairment. It only does so when the canal is narrow and there is retention of debris deep in the canal. Sometimes the tympanic membrane itself is involved, and becomes oedematous and less efficient at transferring sound.

Acute otitis media

Otalgia in association with pyrexia affects more than 50 per cent of infants and young children at some time in their lives. In many countries such children are managed by primary care physicians rather than by otolaryngologists or paediatricians. Acute otitis media is dominant in the differential diagnosis but is perhaps over-diagnosed because otoscopy, the key to diagnosis, can be difficult.

Acute otitis media is an infection of the middle ear mucosa, usually initiated by a viral upper respiratory tract infection affecting the Eustachian tube. This will initially create negative middle ear pressure and retention of middle ear fluid. In some, this becomes secondarily infected with upper respiratory tract bacteria, often *H. influenzae* in older children, and pus collects in the middle ear. The earlier stages of this process will also cause otalgia and be associated with fever. Otalgia will be reported by children that can communicate but in children that cannot it is inferred by indirect signs such as protecting or rubbing the ear. Otalgia can also be caused by teething or sore throats because of referred pain. Children of this age can also be feverish because of a chest or urinary infection.

Otoscopy

In such situations otoscopy is the key to diagnosis. Increased redness or vascularization of the deep canal and the handle of the malleus can be caused by crying or otoscopy itself. In such children the tympanic membrane is normal. With the development of negative middle ear pressure and the retention of middle ear fluid, the pars tensa becomes dull, often inflamed and can be retracted. When pus accumulates, the pars tensa becomes even more inflamed and bulges. Finally, the positive middle ear pressure may be such that the pars tensa perforates and the pus discharges. Pneumatic otoscopy is recommended by some as a means of excluding the diagnosis, as a mobile pars tensa excludes acute otitis media.

Otitis media with effusion

Various terms are used to describe this condition, such as serous otitis media, secretory otitis media, non-purulent otitis media, chronic non-suppurative otitis media and glue ear. This is because the aetiopathology of otitis media with effusion (OME) is uncertain but most would agree that it is the retention within the middle ear space and mastoid air cell system of a non-purulent fluid, associated with chronic inflammatory changes of the middle ear and Eustachian tube mucosa.

OME primarily presents in children between the ages of 2 and 7 years and further discussion of the condition, its monitoring and management in children is left to Chapter 13. Its management in adults is discussed on p. 104. This section discusses diagnosis.

OME is not an easy diagnosis to make but most otologists would consider that otoscopic examination is fairly reliable in detecting the condition. Accepting that there will be occasions when otoscopy is not possible, such as in a screaming child or when there is wax present, how reliable is it and is tympanometry a valuable alternative?

Otoscopy

Clinicians will vary in their otoscopic ability to diagnose otitis media with effusion but the overall 'hit rate' appears to be remarkably poor. In some studies, where it can be assumed that the children were considered to have otoscopic otitis media with effusion prior to surgery, ~ 40 per cent had no middle ear fluid at myringotomy (Haughton, 1977; Orchik, 1978). Allowing for the possibility that in some the fluid may have been displaced by the nitrous oxide anaesthesia, this is an exceedingly high false-positive diagnosis rate for middle ear fluid. What the false-negative rate is in failing to detect middle ear fluid is difficult to ascertain, as clinicians are unlikely to perform a myringotomy if they do not suspect middle ear fluid.

It is possible to improve on the ability to detect middle ear fluid by making a trainee correlate his otoscopic findings with the surgical ones but even then otoscopy is not as accurate as might be hoped. Before a clinician is allowed to participate in one of the Pittsburgh Otitis Media Centre studies, he has to demonstrate that he can minimize his rate of false-positive diagnosis of middle ear fluid to 10 per cent and his false-negative rate (i.e. he fails to detect fluid) to 20 per cent (Stool and Flaherty, 1983).

In such ears it is strongly recommended that an operating microscope, along with a Siegle's speculum with a plain glass lens, be used to evaluate the appearance and mobility of different parts of the pars tensa and flaccida. The otoscopic findings in otitis media with effusion are variable. First the tympanic membrane may be bulging, be in a normal position or be retracted. Its mobility can vary, depending on whether or not there is air as well as fluid in the middle ear and whether there are adhesions. A mobile tympanic membrane does not exclude, nor does immobility imply, otitis media with effusion, but it is a helpful pointer. The tympanic membrane may be tightly indrawn or wrinkled. Its colour has been described as yellowish or bluish. The most difficult ear in which to decide whether there is still middle ear fluid is one where the tympanic membrane has become adherent to the promontory or the long process of the incus.

Tympanometry

Several authors have compared the findings at myringotomy with the tympanogram type (see Figure 4.2) recorded immediately prior to surgery. The practical difficulty with this is that if no fluid is found, it could be claimed that it has drained down the Eustachian tube or into the mastoid air cells since the time of the examination. On the other hand, if fluid is found at operation it is unlikely to have developed since the time of examination. Perhaps the best findings to date are those from Finitzo et al. (1992) (Table 4.2). In their surgical series, where 70

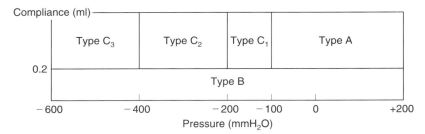

Figure 4.2 Classification of tympanogram types according to Jerger (modification)

per cent of ears had OME, a type B tympanogram had a positive predictive value of 96 per cent. This is superior to their data on otoscopy, including pneumatic otoscopy. Type A and type C tympanograms had a negative predictive value of 53 per cent which is not accurate enough to be of practical use.

Chronic otitis media

The diagnosis of chronic otitis media implies a permanent abnormality of the pars tensa or flaccida. In most patients the initiating factors are unknown but are likely to include acute otitis media, otitis media with effusion and surgery, especially grommet insertion.

There is usually little difficulty in diagnosing chronic otitis media once the external auditory canal has been cleansed of debris and any associated otitis externa allowed to settle, which can take several visits. There is usually no need to give the patient an anaesthetic to clean out the ear to assess the pathology, except perhaps in children. There are several classifications of chronic otitis media but, from the point of view of management, most would agree that three decisions have to be made:

- Are the pars tensa and flaccida intact?
- Is the disease active or inactive?
- If active, is the inflammation confined to the

mucosa or is there squamous epithelium involved as well? In other words, is there a cholesteatoma?

Once the above decisions have been made, the chronic otitis media can be classified as being one of the following types.

Healed chronic otitis media

If the tympanic membrane and pars flaccida are intact and in their normal positions, the disease can be considered healed and unlikely to become active. However, there may be a hearing impairment due to ossicular chain disruption or tympanosclerosis of the tympanic membrane or ossicles.

The best way of confirming that the tympanic membrane is intact is by pneumatic otoscopy, when it will be seen to be mobile. An alternative is to perform tympanometry. When a defect is present the most usual result is a flat tympanogram with a high compliance value which represents the combined volume of the canal and the middle ear space (*Figure 4.3*). The less frequent alternative is that the Eustachian tube allows the air to escape and a seal cannot be obtained.

Inactive chronic otitis media

Here there is either a permanent perforation of the pars tensa or a retracted area in the middle

Table 4.2 Sensitivity and specificity of tympanometry in identifying OME. For definition of B and C_2 tympanograms see Figure 4.2

	Sensitivity	Specificity	PPV	NPV
B versus rest	57	93	96	47
B + C_2 versus rest	88	73	66	53
Otoscopy	93	58	84	77

PPV = positive predictive value; NPV = negative predictive value
(After Finitzo *et al.*, 1992)

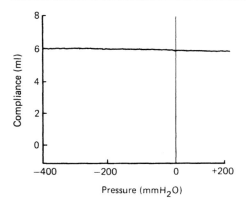

Figure 4.3 Tympanogram in chronic otitis media when there is a tympanic membrane defect

ear or attic. At the time of examination there is no evidence of inflammation ('activity').

In such an ear there are two main concerns, namely any associated hearing impairment and the possibility of future activity. The likelihood of the latter occurring in an ear that is inactive is unknown. It is usually considered that, provided drainage of mucus from the middle ear and mastoid spaces past the ossicles to the Eustachian tube is occurring and there is free exit of epithelial debris from any retracted area, future activity is unlikely. Although advice is often given to avoid water getting into the ears, there is no evidence that this increases the likelihood of activity developing.

Active chronic otitis media

An ear is active if there is pooling of secretions, either mucopus or mucus, in the middle ear or external auditory canal. Provided that all debris is removed from the ear and every part examined there should be little difficulty in deciding if an ear is active or not. The inexperienced often neglect what they think is a piece of wax postero-superiorly in the attic region. This is often not wax but dried pus overlying active disease. As such it is important to remove it to fully examine the pars flaccida.

It is not necessary that the patient has noticed an aural discharge for an ear to be active. It all depends on the volume of the secretions and whether they can drain down the Eustachian tube. Consequently, the length of time a patient has had a discharging ear is not a reliable indicator of the duration of activity.

There are two main variants of activity, the

first being where the inflammation is primarily of the mucosa of the middle ear, antrum and mastoid air cells. This type of disease can be referred to as active, mucosal disease. The second type is where, in addition to the mucosal inflammation, there is a retracted pocket of squamous epithelium filled with epithelial debris; that is a cholesteatoma.

Many otologists would consider it to be particularly important to identify a cholesteatoma because it would be more likely to be associated with life-threatening complications such as an intracranial abscess. The relative chances of complications occurring in mucosal as opposed to cholesteatomatous disease have not been defined, mainly because of the difficulty of assessing the incidence of the two main types of active chronic otitis media in the community. What can be done is to analyse the incidence of cholesteatomatous disease against mucosal disease in patients that present medically (*Table 4.3*).

Complications can be categorized in different ways such as intracranial and extracranial but for clinical practice it is better to think of them in terms of likelihood of occurrence. This is particularly helpful when considering management. A conductive hearing impairment is the commonest complication. Labyrinthitis and sensorineural impairment are not uncommon whilst facial nerve palsy, meningitis, intracranial abscess and lateral sinus thrombosis are thankfully rare. This order of rank is based upon clinical reports rather than hard scientific evidence. The only incidence data are on intracranial abscesses associated with active chronic otitis media. In the UK the chances of active chronic otitis media causing an intracranial abscess are 1 in 10,000 per year

Table 4.3 Relative risks of complications occurring in ears with cholesteatoma compared to those with active mucosal disease

Complication	Cholesteatoma versus mucosal disease
Conductive impairment	No difference[1]
Sensorineural impairment	No difference[1]
Labyrinthitis	Not known
Facial nerve palsy	Mucosal commoner[2]
Meningitis	Mucosal commoner[2]
Intracranial abscess	No difference[2,3]
Lateral sinus thrombosis	No difference[2]

[1]Glasgow Royal Infirmary (GRI) data; [2]Singh and Maharaj (1993); [3]Nunez and Browning (1989)

(Nunez and Browning, 1989). Taken over a lifetime the chances are greater, so that a patient aged 20 has a 1 in 167 chance over the next 60 years of developing an intracranial abscess.

Table 4.3 lists the complications and the relative likelihood of them occurring in cholesteatomatous ears against those with mucosal disease, as evaluated from the literature. As can be seen, there is no evidence that non-cholesteatomatous ears are 'safe'. Surgery is not without its risks and indeed can result in the same complications as the disease process itself. Again, the relative risks, especially in the hands of the average surgeon, are not known, which makes it extremely difficult to assess the advantages of surgery in preventing complications.

It would be helpful if radiology could assess the extent and type of activity. Radiology can identify anatomical defects in the temporal bone provided they are big enough and the correct view has been taken. For example, it is possible to identify defects in the attic but radiology cannot determine the cause. Such defects can be caused by mucosal disease, cholesteatoma or surgery. The ability of mucosal disease to cause bone erosion cannot be doubted because ossicular chain disruption is so frequently associated with it. Radiology will determine what the bony anatomy of a particular temporal bone is but it is unlikely to distinguish mucosal disease from cholesteatoma. Such comments apply to standard X-rays, CT scans and MRI. Radiology is often used to ascertain whether the mastoid air cell system is sclerotic but this will almost invariably be the case if the disease process has been present for any length of time.

Otosclerosis

Otoscopy

Otosclerosis is a diagnosis made by exclusion of other common causes of a conductive defect. When the tympanic membrane is normal in appearance the only alternative diagnoses to be considered are malleus head fixation, congenital middle ear abnormalities and traumatic ossicular chain discontinuity. In comparison to otosclerosis these are uncommon, but it would be valuable to be able to diagnose otosclerosis apart from using surgical explora-

tion of the middle ear. In some ears with otosclerosis, a pink (flamingo) flush may be seen through the tympanic membrane but this is a relatively uncommon finding and is subject to considerable observer error.

Tympanometry

It might be expected that the compliance in ears with otosclerosis would be lower than normal because of decreased mobility of the ossicular chain, whilst the compliance in ears with ossicular discontinuity would be higher. This hypothesis has been studied by several investigators including Jerger *et al.* (1974) (see *Table 4.4*).

When compared with normal ears, those with otosclerosis have a lower mean compliance but there is considerable overlap in the levels as is evident from the 10th and 90th percentiles. Because of this it has been calculated that in a clinic population the false-positive and false-negative rates are unacceptably high (Browning *et al.*, 1985). If the level of compliance is taken which would correctly diagnose the majority (90 per cent) of ears with otosclerosis, then 88 per cent of normal ears would be incorrectly diagnosed as having the condition. Alternatively, if the level of compliance is taken which would correctly diagnose the majority (90 per cent) of normal ears, then 62 per cent of otosclerotic ears would be incorrectly classed as normal. Thus tympanometry has no value in the diagnosis of otosclerosis in an individual patient.

Ossicular chain disruption

Disruption of the ossicular chain, as a result of trauma, is relatively uncommon and most individuals will clearly relate their hearing impairment to the head injury. The tympanic

Table 4.4 Compliance in otosclerosis and ossicular discontinuity in comparison with the normal state

Pathology	n	Mean compliance	Percentiles	
			10th	*90th*
Otosclerosis	95	0.4	0.1	1.0
Discontinuity	19	1.9	0.8	> 3.7
Normal	825	0.7	0.4	1.3

(After Jerger *et al.*, 1974)

membrane will be normal so, in the presence of a conductive hearing impairment, the main alternative diagnosis is otosclerosis. Unfortunately, tympanometry is of no value because of the reasons discussed above.

Fortunately the distinction between ossicular disruption and otosclerosis does not really matter, because the decision as to whether to operate will depend on the patient's disability. If surgery is decided upon, it is hoped that the otologist would be sufficiently skilled to correct whatever abnormality was found at tympanotomy.

Congenital middle ear abnormalities

In adults previously unrecognized middle ear abnormalities are rare in comparison with the other causes of middle ear defect. If there are no congenital stigmata and the external auditory canal is normal, the diagnosis is usually made at surgery for what, up till then, would be thought to be otosclerosis. At this stage whether or not an attempt is made to correct the defect depends on what is found and the expertise of the surgeon.

Identification of a conductive defect

Otoscopy

If middle ear disease is diagnosed by otoscopy, the sound conduction mechanism will be affected and there will be a conductive hearing impairment. Under these circumstances, what one wants to know is its magnitude, and the only way of ascertaining this is by pure-tone audiometry.

Rinne tuning fork test

Tuning fork tests are the traditional clinical method of detecting a conductive defect. There are even some clinicians who use tuning fork tests as a screening method for deciding whether to carry out bone-conduction (b-c) testing. They do this because of the difficulties in performing and interpreting bone-conduction thresholds. Such reliance on tuning fork tests is not justified as discussed earlier (see p. 11 and Browning, 1987). As such, there is no point in doing a Rinne test in ears which are abnormal on otoscopy because the conduction mechanism will be abnormal. In ears that are otoscopically normal and in which a hearing impairment is present, a Rinne negative result (bone conduction louder than air conduction) indicates otosclerosis with an air–bone gap of 10 dB or greater with a 95 per cent degree of confidence. On the other hand,

a Rinne positive result does not help, as there could still be an air–bone gap of up to 30 dB due to otosclerosis.

Pure-tone audiometry

Conductive defects are best identified by the presence of an air–bone gap on a pure tone audiogram and this is the accepted 'gold standard' against which everything else is compared. Unfortunately experienced otologists will recall individuals who had no air–bone gap but in whom there ought to have been a conductive defect because of the presence of a tympanic membrane perforation. Equally, occasions will be recalled where there was a sizeable air–bone gap, but no abnormality could be detected at exploratory tympanotomy. The problems of audiometry are even more marked when the magnitude of the air–bone gap is being assessed (for further discussion see p. 42 and 107).

Acoustic reflexes

It is commonly held that in ears with a conductive defect of 15 dB or greater, the acoustic reflexes will be absent. This figure is rather low if the literature is examined. For example, Lutman (1984) analysed the reflex data available from 1778 ears (*Figure 4.4* and *Table 4.5*) randomly selected from the adult British population, and found that only when the air–bone gap was greater than 30 dB was the reflex absent in more than 90 per cent of patients. The commonly mentioned figure of 15 dB is the level at which 50 per cent of ears will not have a reflex but the other 50 per cent will. This is not sufficiently accurate to detect a meaningful air–bone gap. However, an absent reflex does imply an air–bone gap provided the level of the sound stimulus used to elicit a reflex is sufficient in relation to the pure tone threshold in the ear being stimulated. If the threshold is 55 dB HL or less in the stimulated ear then a reflex would be expected to occur, but not necessarily if it was above that level (see *Figure AIV.5* p. 189). So an absent reflex implies an air–bone gap of greater than 5 dB provided the hearing threshold in the stimulated ear was less than 55 dB at that frequency. However, this does not mean that the majority of ears with an air–bone gap greater than 5 dB will have an absent reflex. It is only when the air–bone gap is 30 dB or greater that a reflex will be absent in 90 per cent of ears.

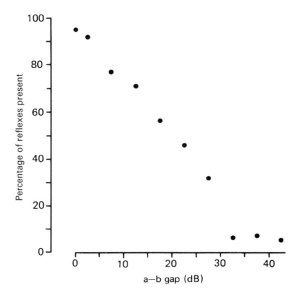

Figure 4.4 Percentage of acoustic reflexes present related to size of air–bone gap (after Lutman, 1984)

Table 4.5 Presence or absence of a contralateral acoustic reflex related to the air–bone gap (mean over 0.5, 1, 2 and 4 kHz)

Air–bone gap (dB)	% Present	% Absent
< 0	95	5
1–5	91	9
6–10	77	23
11–15	71	29
16–20	56	43
21–25	46	54
26–30	32	68
31–35	6	94
36–40	7	93
> 41	6	94

(After Lutman, 1984)

Magnitude of a conductive defect

The air–bone gap

The magnitude of the air–bone gap is the sole method of quantifying the magnitude of a conductive defect, which thus depends on an accurate audiogram.

Validity of pure-tone audiometry

Pure-tone audiometry can, on occasions, be unreliable for several reasons but the majority of these can be controlled. The machines can be calibrated regularly and the tests can be performed in a sound-deadened environment according to a protocol. The headphones and the bone-conduction vibrators can be placed correctly and many subjects are fully co-operative. However, a variable that cannot be controlled for is a fundamental one: the bone-conduction is not a measure of inner ear function and the air conduction cannot invariably be considered to be the same as the threshold would be to free-field sound. Though these aspects have been touched on elsewhere (see pp. 24 and 32) the problems associated with bone-condition thresholds are worth summarizing.

The main problem is that it is sometimes uncertain which ear is being tested. Where the bone vibrator is placed is not too relevant because sound can be transmitted across the skull without being attenuated (see *Table 3.1*, p. 24) The conventional way to overcome this is to mask the non-test ear but the only way to do this is by air conduction. If there is a conductive defect in the non-test ear it may be impossible to mask it sufficiently because there is a limit to the sound output of the machine. This situation is most likely to occur when there is a bilateral conductive defect and it is not infrequent in these circumstances to be unsure of which ear is being tested because of the inability to adequately mask either ear.

The upper limit of the bone-conduction vibrator is ~ 70 dB so that when the patient has a severe or profound impairment (i.e. the air-

conduction thresholds are greater than 70 dB HL) there is no way of determining whether there is a conduction component to the impairment or not (see *Figures 11.1–11.5*, pp. 120–122). Finally, the maximum size an air-bone gap can be is about 60 dB. This is because the bone-conduction vibration inevitably vibrates the air and is heard by air-conduction.

Considering all these possible difficulties with the bone-conduction thresholds, it is easy to understand why the air–bone gap does not invariably detect or accurately quantify the size of a conductive defect.

The Carhart effect

The fact that the bone conduction is not a measure of inner ear function is best explained by reference to two diagrams, one where the conduction mechanism is normal (*Figure 4.5*) and one where it is disrupted (*Figure 4.6*). When the skull is vibrated by bone conduc-

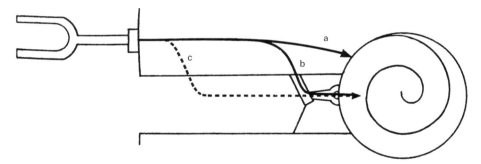

Figure 4.5 The three normal routes (a, b and c) of bone conduction to the inner ear

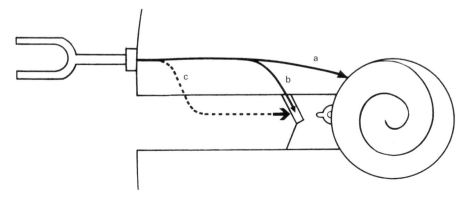

Figure 4.6 In the presence of a conductive defect the osseous route (a) is the only one the bone conduction has to the inner ear

tion, it not only vibrates the cochlea (route a) but it also vibrates the tympanic membrane and ossicular chain (route b) and the air in the external auditory canal (route c). When the ear is normal, bone conduction then has three components (routes a, b and c) and cannot be considered a measure of inner ear function (route a only).

Routes b and c are important as has been shown in experimental work in cats (*Figure 4.7*, after Tonndorf, 1972). When the conduction mechanism is absent (*Figure 4.6*), sound can only go to the cochlea via the bone (route a). If the conduction mechanism is surgically repaired then the components via the canal and ossicular chain (routes b and c) are added to the sound arriving at the cochlea and the bone conduction thresholds will improve.

That the bone conduction thresholds can improve after successful middle ear surgery was first described by Carhart (1950) in patients undergoing fenestration of the lateral semicircular canal for otosclerosis. Since then, many other authors have confirmed this, not only in ears with otosclerosis but in those with chronic otitis media and otitis media with effusion. The magnitude of the effect is greatest at 2 kHz (*Table 4.6*); hence the reason for the Carhart notch (*Figure 4.8*) frequently seen in otosclerosis pre-operatively but also present in all conduction losses. Following successful surgery to restore the sound conduction mechanism, the post-operative bone-conduction

Table 4.6 Carhart effect (dB)

| | kHz | | | |
	0.5	1	2	4
Carhart (1950)	5	10	15	5
Gunderson (1973)	12	12	12	9
Ginsberg *et al.* (1978)	15	17	18	17
Gatehouse and Browning (1982)	5	8	12	5

thresholds will improve at all frequencies, but especially at 2 kHz with the elimination of the notch. Because otosclerotic surgery is more likely to be technically successful than surgery for chronic otitis media, the improvement in bone-conduction thresholds occurs more often following stapes surgery.

There are two main practical implications of the Carhart effect. Firstly, in those with a conductive impairment, the bone-conduction thresholds will be falsely depressed by a mean of 10–15 dB. This, in many instances, will make the patient appear to have a mixed rather than a pure conduction impairment. Secondly, where surgery for otosclerosis is being considered, the post-operative air-conduction thresholds could well be better than the pre-operative bone-conduction thresholds by 10–15 dB. This possibility is also present in surgery for chronic otitis media but is less frequently realized.

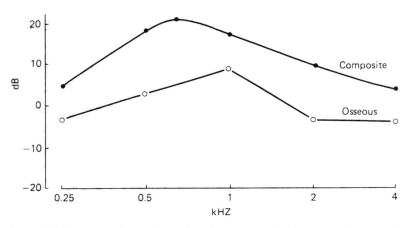

Figure 4.7 The composite cochlear microphonics at various frequencies in cats initiated by stimulating bone conduction. The osseous component is that which arrives at the inner ear via the bone (route a). The remainder is made up of the components arriving at the inner ear via the external auditory canal and the middle ear (routes b and c) (after Tonndorf, 1972)

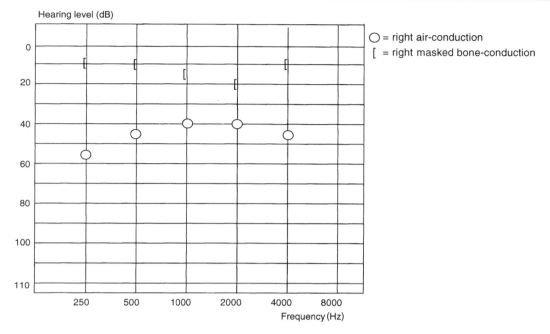

Figure 4.8 Pure tone audiogram of an ear with a conductive impairment. There is a dip in the bone conduction around 2 kHz – the Carhart notch. Note the magnitude of the air–bone gap is greatest at the lower frequencies

Pathophysiological interpretation of the audiogram

Physiology of the tympanic membrane

By strict definition the tympanum is the anatomical term for the tympanic membrane but by common usage it has come to include the middle ear space and the ossicular chain. The tympanic membrane is shaped like a curved cone and is lined by a single layer of squamous epithelium on the canal side and a single layer of mucosa on the middle ear side. In between is a fibrous tissue layer whose collagen fibres are arranged in two main directions. There are radial fibres which run centrally and surround the handle of the malleus and there are circular fibres, a localized concentration of which forms the annulus (*Figure 4.9*). This fibrous tissue layer is the functional key to the tympanic membrane, making it a mobile but relatively inelastic structure which allows the sound pressure to be transmitted along the full length of the handle of the malleus.

Stroboscopic studies at high sound pressure levels have shown that there are two areas of

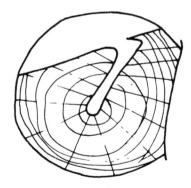

Figure 4.9 Tympanic membrane fibres (after Shimada and Limm, 1971)

tympanic membrane movement, one on either side of the malleus handle (*Figure 4.10*). Because of the physical properties of a curved membrane, the force from the movement of these two areas is transmitted to the malleus handle along its full length (*Figure 4.11*). The malleus handle is, therefore, the key to picking

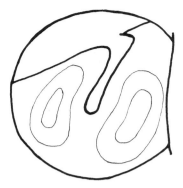

Figure 4.10 Areas of maximum tympanic membrane movement

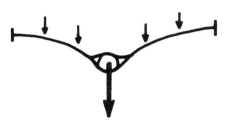

Figure 4.11 Physical properties of the tympanic membrane which transfers all its force of movement to the handle of the malleus along its entire length

up sound energy in a piston system and the suspensory ligaments suspend the ossicular chain to allow movement in a piston-like, rather than a rotatory, manner (*Figure 4.12*). The bodies of the incus and malleus probably act as counterweights to the system, which functions optimally at frequencies up to 4 kHz. Above that, the movement of the tympanic membrane becomes unco-ordinated and the piston system becomes less efficient. When there is a tympanic membrane defect or middle ear pathology the major effect on sound transmission will thus be at the lower as opposed to the

higher frequencies. This is the main reason why an air–bone gap is larger at the low as opposed to the high frequencies (*Figure 4.8*).

Tympanic membrane pathology

Chalk patches are the initial stage and tympanosclerotic plaques the end stage of degeneration of the fibrous collagen layer. Fortunately, chalk patches do not materially affect the sound transmission characteristics of the tympanic membrane because they do not reduce the area or affect the mobility of the tympanic membrane. A tympanosclerotic plaque, on the other hand, can sometimes reduce the membrane's freedom to move if it extends to the annulus, but this is unusual. It is more likely that when there is a large plaque in the tympanic membrane, the ossicular chain will also be fixed by tympanosclerosis and this, rather than the plaque, will be the main cause of the conductive defect.

Let us turn our attention now to a common situation in chronic otitis media, where there is a tympanic membrane defect and the ossicular chain is normal. The magnitude of the conductive defect will primarily relate to the size of the perforation. That this is a real rather than an academic concept has been shown by analysis of the air–bone gap in individuals with a tympanic membrane defect but an intact and normal ossicular chain (*Table 4.7* and *Figure 4.13*).

The larger the perforation the larger is the air–bone gap up to a maximum of ∼ 30 dB. It is wrong to consider that posterior perforations are associated with a larger conductive impairment than anterior perforations because of the loss of the round window baffle effect. Sounds arriving in the same phase and at the same time at the oval and round window will dampen movement of the perilymph but this will occur

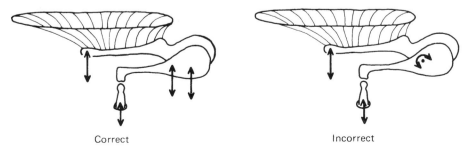

Correct   Incorrect

Figure 4.12 Correct and incorrect direction of ossicular chain movement

Table 4.7 Correlation between size of perforation and air–bone gap

Percentage perforation	Air–bone gap (dB HL ± 1 SD)
0–25	12 ± 7.5
26–50	22 ± 8.5
51–95	28 ± 9.0

(After Austin, 1978)

no matter where the perforation is. The reason why posterior perforations are more often associated with larger air–bone gaps than similarly sized anterior perforations is that the former are more likely to be associated with ossicular chain abnormalities than the latter.

Physiology of the ossicular chain

The ossicular chain is suspended in the middle ear, mainly by its ligaments and the intra-tympanic muscles (*Figure 4.14*). The ligaments are not often considered to be important but dislocation of the incus and its interposition between the stapes and the malleus in a tympanoplasty is not as inherently stable as a normal ossicular chain (*Figure 4.15*). Hence, many simply heighten the stapes with an ossicle or cartilage to make direct contact with the tympanic membrane (*Figure 4.16*) to create a piston system. This, because of its stability, often closes the air–bone gap as much as more complicated ossiculoplasty procedures.

Many would consider that the function of the

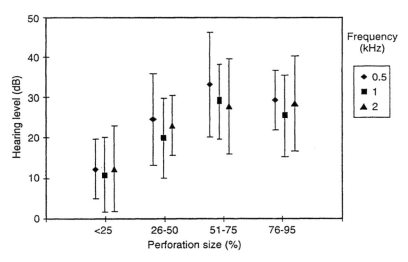

Figure 4.13 Mean air–bone gap at 0.5, 1 and 2 kHz related to the size of the perforation in ears with an intact and mobile ossicular chain. Bars indicate ± 1 SD (after Austin, 1978)

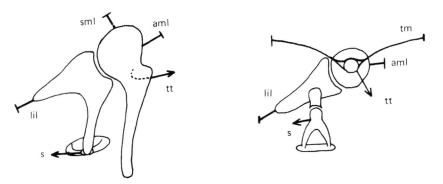

Figure 4.14 Ossicular chain suspension. aml = anterior malleolar ligament; lil = lateral incudal ligament; s = stapedius muscle; sml = superior malleolar ligament; tm = tympanic membrane; tt = tensor tympani

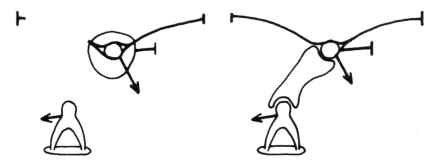

Figure 4.15 Relative instability of an incus interposition due to the direction of pull of the middle ear muscles

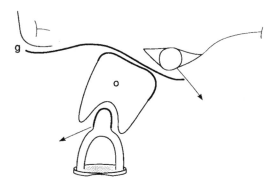

Figure 4.16 Piston system recreated in ossiculoplasty by heightening the stapes. g = graft; o = repositioned ossicle

stapedius and tensor tympani muscles is to prevent the inner ear being damaged by external noise but this is seriously doubted for several reasons:

- Reflex contraction of the middle ear muscles in response to noise only attenuates the lower frequencies.
- The contraction occurs too slowly to be of value for impulse noise.
- High continuous noise levels seldom occur in nature but they do in 'civilized' societies. Although such noise will initially be attenuated by the reflexes, these fatigue with time and become less effective.
- In humans, the tensor tympani does not contract in response to sound.

What their exact role is, is uncertain, but they could be an attenuator of internally produced sound from the vocal tract. Their surgical division, as in stapedectomy or tympanoplasty, is likely to be of little consequence.

In man the incudo-malleolar joint would appear to have no function apart from holding the two bones together as there is no movement at the joint. Indeed, in many rodents there is no joint and the malleus and incus are one bone. The incudo-stapedial joint, on the other hand, functions as a true synovial joint.

The function of the tympanum is to transmit sounds from the external auditory canal to the perilymph in the inner ear. Fluids are much less compressible than air and, in order to compensate for what otherwise would be a loss of sound energy, the conduction mechanism acts as a piston system. The area of the tympanic membrane is nearly 20 times the area of the stapes footplate and this overcomes the resistance to movement of fluid in the middle ear compared to air.

How the ossicular chain functions in this piston system is important to understand, especially if it is hoped to reconstruct it in ears damaged by chronic otitis media. There is a small lever component (*Figure 4.12*, incorrect example) but its contribution is small.

Ossicular chain pathology

The two main pathologies that affect the ossicles are otosclerosis and chronic otitis media. In clinical otosclerosis, the footplate can become progressively fixed by obliteration of the fibrous joint starting anteriorly. The air–bone gap can thus gradually increase up to a maximum of 60 dB. The reason why an air–bone gap of greater than 60 dB is not possible is because 60 dB above the bone-conduction thresholds of the audiometer will vibrate the skull sufficiently by air conduction for it to be heard by bone conduction.

In chronic otitis media, apart from tympanic membrane pathology, the ossicular chain can be affected to various degrees either by tympanosclerosis or necrosis. The magnitude of the air–bone gap, along with otoscopic assessment of the ossicular chain, can give some indication of the likely pathology but a final assessment can only be made at surgery when the chain can be more fully examined. This is because in many instances there are adhesions between the promontory and the tympanic membrane and ossicles. Alternatively, the tympanic membrane can be retracted on to the remaining parts of the chain, such as the long process of the incus and the stapes superstructure. Thus, when the ossicular chain is disrupted the size of the air–bone gap can vary from 0 dB up to a maximum of ~ 60 dB. Naturally the size of the air–bone gap is unrelated to where the disruption in the chain is, disruption of the incudo-stapedial joint being able to cause as large an air–bone gap as total absence of the ossicular chain.

The general rule must be that in chronic otitis media a conductive hearing impairment of up to 15 dB can be explained by a perforation. An impairment of between 15 and 30 dB may be explained by a perforation if it affects more than 25 per cent of the tympanic membrane, but there may also be ossicular chain problems. In these circumstances, it is a matter of debate whether it is better, surgically, to leave the ossicular chain and the adhesions alone or to attempt to reconstruct the ossicular chain. If the conductive hearing impairment is greater than 40 dB there almost certainly will be ossicular chain problems and a myringoplasty alone is unlikely to resolve the hearing problem.

■ Conclusions

• Otoscopy will identify the majority of conditions of the external auditory canal and middle ear. The main exception to this is otosclerosis.
• Wax frequently needs to be removed to perform otoscopy.
• Wax is infrequently a cause of a hearing impairment unless it is impacted deep in the canal.
• Otitis externa is usually associated with a mild impairment.
• Acute otitis media is mainly a condition of infants and young children. Its otoscopic diagnosis can be difficult and follow-up is important to identify the small proportion of cases that progress to otitis media with effusion.
• Otitis media with effusion is the commonest cause for a hearing impairment in young children. Its otoscopic diagnosis can be difficult but can be aided by tympanometry.
• Chronic otitis media is primarily a condition of adults, affecting about 6 per cent of the UK adult population. At any one time the ear may be active or inactive and the condition may be pathologically associated with mucosal disease or a cholesteatoma (squamous disease).
• Otosclerosis is the presumptive diagnosis in those with a normal tympanic membrane associated with a conductive hearing impairment. It affects about 2 per cent of adults. Tympanometry is of no value in confirming the diagnosis.
• The air–bone gap in pure tone audiometry is the sole means of assessing the magnitude of a conductive defect. It is important to have accurate bone-conduction thresholds to assess this. Their interpretation also requires knowledge of what they are a measure of.
• Tuning fork tests and acoustic reflexes have no role when there is otoscopic evidence of pathology that can cause a conductive defect.
• A knowledge of the physiology of sound conduction is essential to correlate otoscopy with the audiogram. This is particularly important if reconstructive surgery is being considered.

Further reading

Browning, G.G. (1997). Aetiopathology of inflammatory conditions of the external and middle ear. In *Otology*, Vol. 3, Chap. 2, Scott-Brown's Otolaryngology. Butterworth-Heinemann, Oxford.

5 Progressive bilateral sensorineural hearing impairments

By far the commonest type of hearing impairment in the population is a slowly progressive sensorineural defect which affects both ears to the same degree. The prevalence of such impairments increases with age (*Table 5.1*), but it is wrong to think that age is the cause. Most degenerative pathologies, such as cardiovascular disease, become commoner with age, but they are not caused by age. It is simply that as an individual gets older they have had more chance to be exposed to the aetiological factors responsible for a condition. So it is as ridiculous to say that 'the commonest cause of hearing loss is age' as it is to say that 'the commonest cause of myocardial infarction is age'.

The term 'presbycusis' is often used to describe age-related hearing impairments and implies a pathological diagnosis. This is not the case, and indeed it does not warrant a separate classification in the World Health Organization International Classification of Diseases (1977). Presbycusis is the name of a syndrome complex, signifying 'the lessening of the acuteness of hearing that characterizes old age' (*Oxford English Dictionary*) for which the aetiology is unknown. 'Age-related hearing loss' is an alternative term which removes the disease connotation. It is likely that several interacting aetiologies will be identified as the cause. Surprisingly, at this stage in our knowledge, there does not appear to be a familial predisposition to develop an age-related, sensorineural hearing impairment.

Various histological changes have been described in the cochlea in elderly individuals who, prior to death, were known to have an idiopathic sensorineural hearing impairment. Similar changes are present in those with a sensorineural impairment due to factors such as noise, so there is no specific pathology associated with ageing. In the majority, the

Table 5.1 Prevalence of hearing defects in adult British population in the better (BE) and worse (WE) hearing ear overall and in four age categories

| | Overall | | Age bands (years) | | | | | | | |
| | | | 17–30 | | 31–50 | | 51–70 | | 70+ | |
	BE	WE	BE	WE	BE	WE	BE	WE	BE	WE
Normal	81	68	96	86	86	72	73	56	27	25
Conductive	6	13	2	12	9	17	6	12	0	3
Mixed	2	5	1	0	0	2	3	8	9	15
Sensorineural	11	14	0.5	1	4	9	17	23	62	56

(After Browning and Davis, 1983)

cochlea is the initial site of the defect but with time this invariably leads to secondary neuronal degeneration, the end result being a combined sensorineural, rather than a pure sensory or a pure neuronal, impairment.

In an audiology clinic the proportion of patients with a pure sensorineural as opposed to a conductive or mixed impairment is less than in the general population (*Table 5.1*). There are several reasons for this. Sensorineural impairments are commoner in the elderly who expect to develop age-related conditions. They are therefore less likely to consult than younger individuals who are more likely to have a conductive impairment. Patients with a mixed impairment are also likely to consult earlier because the combined defect gives a greater impairment. In such cases it would be wrong to consider the middle ear pathology responsible for the sensorineural impairment, it is just that they frequently co-exist.

Clinical assessment

In an individual with a bilateral sensorineural impairment, clinical assessment has three aims:

- to identify any aetiological factors;
- to assess the degree of disability; and
- to suggest management.

In most patients, attempting to identify the aetiology is likely to be unrewarding as in 94 per cent of patients it is unknown (Browning and Davis, 1983). In 5 per cent noise exposure has an influence and in a further 1 per cent other aetiologies can be implicated. If it is necessary to ascribe a diagnostic label to patients with an idiopathic, sensorineural impairment, they should be considered to have an age-related hearing loss rather than presbycusis.

Identification of aetiological factors

Noise exposure

A noise exposure history in patients with a sensorineural impairment can give unexpected replies. It is surprising how often a 'dear old lady' worked in a factory in her youth. Individuals who have worked in similar noisy environments for the same length of time vary in their susceptibility to damage. Some will have no hearing impairment whereas others will be severely impaired. The reasons for this variation in susceptibility are unknown but there could be a genetic predisposition. It is also likely that the various aetiological factors will have a cumulative and perhaps a synergistic effect, so that in some there will be damage due to other factors and the noise trauma simply makes the impairment more marked.

The thoroughness with which a noise exposure history is taken depends on whether the patient is claiming compensation. In developed countries, government legislation and increased awareness in the work-force has meant an increase in the number of such cases. In the United Kingdom there are three main methods of making a claim.

Government compensation

There are some proscribed occupations such as drop forging, shipbuilding and metal working where pneumatic percussion or grinding tools are used. A worker who has been exposed to such noise for at least 20 years and who has a pure tone average of 50 dB HL or worse over 1, 2 and 3 kHz in his better hearing ear is compensated. Understandably there is pressure to extend this cover to other industries and to lower the level of hearing loss at which compensation becomes payable.

Armed forces

Certain pensions are payable for noise-induced hearing loss caused by gun-fire, both in peacetime and at war. These pensions are administered by the Ministry of Defence so details are not available as to how a decision is made.

Common law

It is possible under common law for anyone exposed to noise to claim compensation from the party responsible for the noise. Currently the majority of claims are under common law and are usually settled out of court. In arriving at a settlement, many factors are taken into consideration, not least of which is the medical opinion as to whether the patient's hearing impairment is likely to have been caused by noise. This opinion is usually given after comparing the noise exposure history with the claimant's pure tone audiogram.

Assessment of noise exposure

There are three types of noise exposure to enquire about: employment, gun-fire and social, the details enquired about in each being different but following the general format:

- Was there any noise exposure?
- If yes to the above, was ear protection worn?
- And how much exposure was there?

Was there employment exposure?

The first question usually is 'What was the noisiest job you have ever worked in?'. The level of noise exposure of any specific job can then be estimated from tables of the commoner noisy occupations (*Table 5.2*). The figures in such tables are approximate and should be confirmed by asking how close a worker had to be and what level of voice had to be used to communicate with fellow workers. A further table (*Table 5.3*) is then consulted to allow a second estimation of the noise level to be made. The ideal is to measure the actual noise levels but this is impracticable in most instances because the factory has often shut down or made modifications to comply with modern standards. Noise exposure levels are measured in dB A, which is similar but not identical to dB HL. It is generally considered that noise exposure at levels of less than 85 dB A are insignificant and can be discounted. If the level of noise exposure in the noisiest job a claimant has had is greater than 85 dB A, any other noisy jobs they may have had are enquired about in the same way.

Was ear protection worn?

The fact that ear protection devices are provided does not mean that they are worn. Ear-

Table 5.2 Occupational noise exposure*

Occupation type	Noise levels (dB A)
Agricultural machinery (e.g. tractor)	93
Aviation aircrew (combat jet)	105
Bottling, bottle cleaning and canning	96
Fabrication (metal)	90
Food industry	87
Iron and steel working	
(blast furnaces, blacksmith, heavy hammering)	99
(heavy forging)	102
(plating and press-shops)	96
Lumber work	99
Paper manufacture	90
Printing	93
Road drilling	96
Seamen (boiler room, other engines)	90
Shipbuilding (near boilermaking, caulking, rust-scaling, riveting)	100
Textiles (weaving and spinning)	99
Tobacco (cigarette manufacturing machinery)	93
Transportation (diesel, heavy goods vehicles)	93
Woodworking/sawmill	90

*These examples are a guide to equivalent continuous noise levels. The levels given are typical ones; individual exposures can be +10 to −20 dB A different

Table 5.3 Noise exposure levels (dB A) as estimated from distance and voice levels at which conversation was possible

| | Distance apart to be heard | | |
	4 feet	2 feet	Close to ear
Normal voice	< 81	–	–
Raised voice	87	–	–
Very loud voice	93	–	–
Shouting	99	105	–
Impossible			> 110

muffs can be uncomfortable and many use them only when the task is particularly noisy. The wearing of muffs also makes it more difficult to communicate with fellow workers. Radio communication is an expensive but effective solution to this. So it is insufficient to ask if protection was worn: the percentage of time it was used during the period of noise exposure must be ascertained.

In addition, it is essential to find out what type of protection it was, in case it was not real protection. Cotton wool plugs, even if coated with Vaseline, are useless. Commercial products vary in their effectiveness and are more efficient at some frequencies than others. *Table 5.4* is a list of the mean attenuation such products give, provided they are correctly worn. These attenuation figures are then subtracted from the estimated noise exposure level. In most instances the wearing of ear protection of any type reduces the exposure level to below 85 dB A and that particular exposure can, thereafter, be discounted.

If protection has been worn only part of the time, the number of years of exposure is amended accordingly.

How much exposure?

The number of years spent in each noisy job is ascertained. The next question is to find out on average what proportion of the day, week and year was actually spent in the noise. It is perhaps easier, especially if ear protection has been worn, to split the job into several parts and calculate the number of years out of the total that were spent at each noise level.

In the majority of instances, performing such a calculation is relatively easy. Detailed calculations are only necessary when someone has been in many different jobs and is claiming compensation for one or more of them, when an apportionment has to be made.

Was there gun-fire exposure?

The simple question here is 'Have you ever fired a gun and if so what type?'. For the militarily inexperienced the various types of gun can be confusing but it is the bore (size) of the barrel that counts. In terms of noise exposure, airguns and small bore (.22) rifles and pistols can be discounted. Thereafter, guns can be classified as rifles (larger than .22) or big guns (bigger than a rifle).

Was ear protection worn?
If ear protection was worn, gun-fire exposure can be discounted. Whether ear protection was available depends on the era in which the exposure occurred. Protection has been provided for many years for all 'big' guns but not necessarily in active service. It is relatively recently that ear protection has been issued in the Forces on practice rifle ranges. Again it is only recently that sportsmen have worn protection.

How much exposure?
This is assessed on the number of rounds that have been fired. It is not necessary, and indeed it is impossible, to get this figure accurately for each type of gun that may have been fired. However, it is usually possible to get the patient to state whether the number is in the tens, hundreds, thousands or tens of thousands of rounds.

Was there social exposure?

Though many individuals use power tools and others go to dance clubs, the cumulative

Table 5.4 Mean attenuation of ear defenders

Type	Attenuation (dB)
Ear muffs	24
Ear plugs	
'EAR'	21
Others	15

exposure is hardly ever sufficient to cause damage. The noise levels at clubs are likely to be at least 99 dB A, but for this to be as likely to cause damage as a job at 99 dB A would require someone to go seven times a week, for 6 hours each time for 50 weeks in the year. Few could keep this up on a social or even a professional basis. Should, on rare occasions, such a fanatic be encountered, exposure can be calculated as for employment exposure.

Calculation of noise immission level

At this stage the amount and duration of the exposure in each of the three classes has been calculated. It is now simply a matter of looking up the appropriate tables (Robinson and Shipton, 1977) which calculate what the NIL (noise immission level) is for a given level of noise exposure and for a given number of years. Such calculations are only really necessary in legal cases or for research purposes.

Comparison with normal thresholds

Having confirmed that an individual has been materially exposed to noise, a comparison should be made of their thresholds with the hearing in individuals matched for age, sex and socio-economic group who have not been exposed to noise. Such data for the UK population are available in various tables (Davis, 1995) based on the MRC National Study of Hearing. The best tables to use are those where individuals with an air–bone gap have been excluded. Table 5.5 shows such a table for the better hearing ear in males in manual occupations between the ages of 51 and 60 years.

Ototoxic drugs

Aminoglycoside ototoxicity usually occurs rapidly over a few days and, as it is most often noticed by the patient at the time, it is usually managed as for a sudden hearing loss (see p. 70). It is rare to make a diagnosis of aminoglycoside ototoxicity some time after it has occurred. Similar comments apply to diuretics and antimitotic drugs.

The only drugs that are commonly prescribed which might cause a progressive, rather than sudden, loss are salicylates and beta-blockers. The impairment caused by salicylates is reversible which makes the diagnosis easy. If a patient with a sensorineural impairment is on a beta-blocker it is probably worth changing to an alternative prescription. Unfortunately, in such a patient the most likely cause is not the drug but the underlying arteriosclerosis, so an improvement in hearing cannot be expected.

General disease

Though many diseases have been postulated to cause a sensorineural impairment, the high prevalence of hearing impairment in the population has to be controlled for when studying the incidence in a specific disease. Before a disease can be considered unequivocally to cause a sensorineural hearing impairment, the following evidence would have to be presented:

- Increased incidence of hearing impairment in individuals with the disease compared with controls.
- Severity of hearing impairment related to the duration and/or the severity of the disease.
- Satisfactory treatment of the disease stops the hearing impairment from progressing or even improves it.

Table 5.6 summarizes the current evidence with respect to various diseases.

Diabetes

Though many papers do not show an increased incidence of sensorineural hearing impairment in patients with diabetes, Tay et al. (1995) fairly convincingly shows this to be the case against three different control populations. The severity of the hearing loss was related to the duration of diabetes but surprisingly not with the severity of the diabetes as evidenced by diabetic retinopathy.

Syphilis

Sensorineural hearing loss certainly occurs in congenital syphilis but is rare in early or late acquired syphilis. In an individual with a

Table 5.5 UK National Study of hearing pure tone thresholds

Sample = no noise or ABG > 0; ear = better ear; age group = 51–60 years; occupational group = manual; gender = male

	Single frequency (kHz)								Combined frequency (kHz)					
	0.250	0.500	1	2	3	4	6	8	4FA	3FA	HFA	LFA	A123	A124
Mean	13.0	10.2	10.4	13.4	27.4	32.5	45.6	44.4	16.6	11.3	40.8	11.2	17.1	18.8
SD	7.3	13.2	11.7	14.8	13.9	13.0	13.7	13.8	11.8	12.5	11.6	10.3	12.4	12.1
Lower CI	10.8	7.5	7.2	9.8	22.9	27.6	42.5	39.5	13.8	8.7	37.2	8.9	13.9	15.5
Upper CI	15.2	13.0	13.7	16.9	31.9	37.4	48.6	49.3	19.5	14.0	44.4	13.6	20.2	22.1
P05	-1.0	0.0	-7.0	-6.0	10.0	13.0	23.0	23.0	6.0	-2.7	22.3	0.7	5.3	6.3
P10	5.0	0.0	0.0	0.0	14.0	20.0	30.0	25.0	7.2	2.0	27.3	3.7	8.7	9.7
P15	9.0	1.0	1.0	4.0	14.0	20.0	30.0	26.0	7.8	2.3	28.7	4.0	9.7	10.3
P20	10.0	1.0	3.0	4.0	17.0	21.0	31.0	29.0	7.8	2.3	28.7	4.0	10.0	10.3
P25	11.0	2.0	3.0	5.0	18.0	22.0	34.0	32.0	9.0	4.7	32.3	4.3	10.0	10.3
P50	14.0	10.0	9.0	10.0	24.0	29.0	45.0	43.0	13.2	10.3	40.0	10.0	11.7	14.0
P75	16.0	15.0	15.0	20.0	34.0	49.0	60.0	63.0	22.2	15.7	55.0	16.0	22.7	28.0
P80	20.0	16.0	15.0	28.0	35.0	50.0	61.0	65.0	27.8	18.7	55.0	17.7	26.7	33.0
P85	23.0	21.0	21.0	30.0	37.0	55.0	63.0	67.0	28.5	19.3	56.3	18.7	21.7	33.0
P90	23.0	21.0	21.0	36.0	56.0	56.0	63.0	69.0	28.8	24.0	58.7	18.7	33.7	33.3
P95	36.0	55.0	50.0	55.0	57.0	56.0	68.0	69.0	54.0	53.3	60.0	46.3	54.0	53.7
N	19	19	19	19	19	19	19	19	19	19	19	19	19	19
Deft	47.2	78.2	56.3	75.4	75.6	63.9	77.3	66.3	71.5	71.6	72.3	61.7	73.4	68.2
Bias	199.7	-195.9	-99.1	-149.8	-43.8	-56.5	-111.5	-144.3	-125.3	-148.3	-104.1	-164.9	-97.6	-101.8

4FA = average over 0.5, 1, 2 and 4 kHz; 3FA = average over 0.5, 1 and 2 kHz; HFA = average over 4, 6 and 8 kHz; LFA = average over 0.250, 0.5 and 1 kHz; A123 = average over 1, 2, and 3 kHz; A124 = average over 1, 2 and 4 kHz

(After Davis, 1995)

Table 5.6 Evidence relating sensorineural hearing impairment to various diseases

	Incidence	Severity	Treatment effective
Diabetes	Yes	Yes	No
Paget's disease	Yes	Yes	No
Cardiovascular disease	?	NA	NA
Hypertension	?	?	NA
Myxoedema	?	No	?
Rheumatoid arthritis	NA	No	NA
Acquired syphilis	No	Yes	?

No = evidence does not support a relationship or an effect; ? = conflicting evidence; NA = evidence not available

sudden sensorineural hearing impairment, syphilitic meningitis in the early stages of an acquired infection could be responsible, though it is usual to have other symptoms of meningitis. In late acquired syphilis a hearing impairment is unlikely unless neurosyphilis has developed. A positive serological test in an individual with a sensorineural impairment should be interpreted with caution as individuals with acquired syphilis are as likely as the general population to develop sensorineural impairments due to other reasons. That this is important to remember is demonstrated by a random survey of the adult population where seven individuals had positive syphilis serology but none had a hearing impairment (MRC National Study of Hearing, personal communication).

There is no doubt that patients with positive syphilis serology need to be treated with a substantial course of penicillin and perhaps steroids in addition. It is doubtful whether such treatment has any effect on the hearing.

Paget's disease

In theory Paget's disease could cause a conductive impairment by affecting the ossicles and a sensorineural impairment by surrounding the cochlea or narrowing the external auditory canal. Well-controlled studies are few but there is evidence from a recent study with two different control groups that in those with radiological involvement of the skull with Paget's disease there is an increased incidence of sensorineural but not conductive hearing impairment (Moeller et al., 1997).

Cardiovascular disease and hypertension

Despite the high prevalence of vascular disease in the population and a 'gut feeling' that it cannot be good for the inner ear, there are surprisingly few controlled studies that have looked for a correlation. What evidence there is would support a correlation between hearing impairment and both cardiac disease and hypertension (MRC National Study of Hearing, presentation to the Royal Society of Medicine, 1982, and Gates et al., 1993). Cardiovascular disease can be evident as myocardial ischaemia, stroke or intermittent claudication. The relationship between hearing impairment and stroke is perhaps the strongest (Gates et al., 1993). Predictors of cardiovascular disease such as hyperlipidaemia, though postulated to be associated with raised hearing thresholds, are not as yet proven (Jones, 1997).

Hypothyroidism

Hypothyroid cretins have a high incidence of hearing defects and there is considerable anecdotal evidence that acquired hypothyroidism can also be associated with a hearing impairment, but there is conflicting evidence as to whether elderly patients with myxoedema have a higher incidence of impairment than age-matched controls (Parving et al., 1983; Hall et al., 1985). The effect of treatment with thyroxine is also controversial, some papers reporting improvement and others no change. The overall conclusion must be that the relationship between acquired hypothyroidism and hearing impairment is unknown but any effect there is will be small.

Rheumatoid arthritis

It has been suggested that there might be an increased incidence of both middle and inner ear problems in individuals with rheumatoid arthritis but no controlled studies have been reported. What evidence there is would suggest that if there is a relationship, it is not related to the severity of the arthritis.

Cochlear otosclerosis

Whether otosclerosis can cause inner ear damage when the footplate is not fixed is controversial but the evidence is that it is unlikely. It has been extremely difficult to prove in controlled studies (Browning and Gatehouse, 1984) that when the stapes is fixed (stapedial otosclerosis) the bone-conduction thresholds once amended for the Carhart effect are elevated compared to normal. Even in the papers that purport to demonstrate a difference, the amount that the thresholds are raised by is relatively small (Glorig and Gallo, 1962; Sataloff *et al.*, 1964). Histologically it is rare for the otosclerotic focus to surround the cochlea to any extent if it does not affect the footplate, so though pure cochlear otosclerosis cannot be discounted it is likely to be rare.

It has been suggested, mainly by Valvasorri, that cochlear otosclerosis can be diagnosed radiographically. Other radiologists have not been so confident and what evidence there is would suggest that the radiological abnormalities described are not associated with histological evidence of cochlear otosclerosis.

Assessment of hearing impairment and disability

Pure tone audiometry

The standard routine in most clinics is to ask for a pure tone audiogram. Apart from confirming that there is a bilateral symmetrical hearing impairment, this is of no help in arriving at a diagnosis of the aetiology. The presence of a 'dip' in the audiogram at 3, 4 or 6 kHz does not 'confirm' the diagnosis of noise-induced hearing loss, as many patients who have not been exposed to noise will have dips. Equally, the absence of a 'dip' does not exclude noise trauma as a factor. The slope of the audiogram is also of no help because of the considerable overlap in the shape of the audiogram in different conditions.

The pure tone average helps to predict the likely disability provided the thresholds in the better hearing ear are taken (see p. 105).

Speech audiogram

If this is available, then it may be of value in two ways. In some patients it will describe the hearing impairment more fully than the pure tone audiogram; the optimal discrimination score (ODS) will indicate the overall effect of cochlear, neural and central defects and the half peak level elevation (HPLE) will give some indication of monaural disability (see Appendix V).

Other auditory tests

The use of other audiometric tests to determine whether there is recruitment or tone decay adds little to the diagnosis. The former can be of benefit in hearing aid provision (see p. 83).

Management

The vast majority of individuals will have no identifiable cause for their impairment, so management is of their disability, usually with hearing aids, rather than their pathology. The exception is noise exposure. If this is still occurring and cannot be avoided, ear protection should be worn. If a generalized disease is identified it ought to be managed for its own sake. However, it is very unlikely that this will have any effect on the hearing.

■ Conclusions

• Progressive, bilateral sensorineural impairments are the commonest type of impairment in the adult population.
• The vast majority are of unknown aetiology.
• Noise exposure is the commonest recognized factor.
• In any individual the effect of noise is perhaps less than might be expected and noise by no means affects every individual who has been exposed to it.
• Though the prevalence of bilateral sensorineural impairments increases with age, age itself is not a cause. It is just that most conditions become commoner with advancing years because there has been more chance of exposure to aetiological factors.
• Presbycusis is, therefore, not a diagnosis with a recognized pathology, but a syndrome signifying the gradual deterioration in hearing that often, but by no means invariably, occurs with advancing years.
• Age-related hearing impairment is a better syndrome label.
• There is no proven association between any general disease and bilateral sensorineural hearing impairments apart from diabetes, Paget's disease and neurosyphilis.
• Ototoxic damage from aminoglycosides and diuretics is rare except when there is associated renal damage. It usually presents at the time as a sudden hearing loss. Beta-blockers have been implicated but it could well be the underlying disease process for which these have been given that is responsible rather than the drug itself.

• Ototoxic damage can affect one or both ears.
• Cochlear otosclerosis is a controversial topic but it is unlikely to be a common entity, especially as it has been difficult to prove that stapedial otosclerosis commonly affects the inner ear.
• The shape of the pure tone audiogram has no diagnostic significance in those with a bilateral sensorineural impairment.
• No audiometric test has a role in diagnosing the aetiology.
• The main role of audiometry is to assess disability and aid in management.
• In the majority, the management is of the disability with hearing aids rather than the pathology. The exception is the wearing of ear protection when noise exposure is still occurring.

Further reading

British Association of Otolaryngologists and the British Society of Audiology (1983). Method for assessment of hearing disability. *British Journal of Audiology*, **17**, 203–212.

Davis, A. (1995). *Hearing in Adults*. Whurr Publishers, London.

King, P.F., Coles, R.R.A., Lutman, M.E. and Robinson, D.W. (1992). Assessment of hearing disability. In *Guidelines for Medico-Legal Practice*. Whurr Publishers, London.

Tempest, W. and Bryan, M.E. (1981). Industrial hearing loss: compensation in the United Kingdom. In *Audiology and Audiological Medicine*. Oxford University Press, Oxford, pp. 846–860.

6 Asymmetric sensorineural impairments

Normally the hearing in an individual's two ears is identical. Asymmetric hearing is thus a result of disease affecting only one ear or both ears but to a different degree. As hearing is most frequently assessed by pure tone audiometry, asymmetry is usually defined as a difference between the thresholds in the two ears. A 10 dB or greater difference in the pure tone average is the level most frequently taken, though patients often detect smaller differences. Some consider that an average difference as small as 10 dB is of no diagnostic relevance and prefer to use a difference of 15 or 20 dB. An alternative approach is to look at individual frequencies, where a difference of 20 dB or greater is unlikely to be due to test error. In addition, there is no reason why asymmetry cannot be defined in terms of speech audiometry or any other monaural test. Some clinicians consider unilateral tinnitus in the presence of symmetric pure tone thresholds to be an indicator of asymmetry.

Using a difference between ears of an average 20 dB as the criterion of asymmetry, one-third of individuals in an ORL clinic will have asymmetric air-conduction thresholds (Glasgow Royal Infirmary clinic data) which is considerably higher than in the general population. The reason for this is perhaps the fact that a patient is more likely to notice a unilateral as opposed to a bilateral symmetric impairment because the 'good ear' can be used for comparison.

What difference does the presence of asymmetric air-conduction thresholds make to the initial assessment of a patient? In two-thirds of cases the reason for the asymmetry is the presence of a conductive defect in one or both ears. In the other third the asymmetry is attributable to differences in inner ear function. In a few the asymmetry will be of both the air- and bone-conduction thresholds. So, for example, there is no reason why an individual with otosclerosis or chronic otitis media would be less likely than anyone else to have asymmetric inner ear function due to an acoustic neuroma. It is important therefore to look for asymmetry in the bone-conduction thresholds when a conduction defect is present, but in doing so it is necessary to consider the Carhart effect (see p. 43).

When there is a bilateral conductive defect this will apply equally to both ears so the bone-conduction thresholds can be inspected for asymmetry without correction. When there is a unilateral conductive defect it is only necessary to correct the bone-conduction thresholds. This is most easily done by subtracting 15 dB from the mean bone-conduction threshold on that side. If asymmetric bone-conduction thresholds are then identified it is often suggested that this is because the middle ear disease has also damaged the inner ear. This may sometimes be the case, but in general there is little difference between the amended bone-conduction thresholds in individuals with otosclerosis or chronic otitis media compared with those in the general population (Browning and Gatehouse, 1983; Browning and Gatehouse, 1984).

The next section deals with the diagnostic dilemma posed by asymmetric sensorineural thresholds. The problems that asymmetric thresholds can lead to in masking, disability and management are dealt with in the appropriate sections.

Aetiology

Acoustic neuroma (vestibular schwannoma)

The inexperienced might consider that acoustic neuroma is a likely diagnosis in a patient with asymmetric sensorineural thresholds. This is not the case (*Table 6.1*). The incidence in the population of asymmetric sensorineural thresholds is 0.7 per cent (MRC National Study of Hearing data). In a UK hospital setting where investigation of patients with unilateral or lateralizing otological symptoms is routine, approximately 4–5% of patients will have an acoustic neuroma identified (Swan and Gatehouse, 1991).

In practice then how is an acoustic neuroma detected or, more frequently, excluded? The first task is to consider whether a patient has one of the recognized aetiologies for asymmetric hearing (*Table 6.1*).

Vestibular syndromes

Several vestibular syndromes (e.g. chronic labyrinthitis and Ménière's syndrome) can be associated with asymmetrical sensorineural thresholds. Such patients usually merit investi-

gation as acoustic neuromas are tumours of the vestibular nerve and many have past vestibular symptoms though these are usually minor.

Congenital and childhood infections

Some will know that they have had a poorer hearing ear since childhood. If on testing this is sensorineural in type, the potential aetiologies are congenital, viral (mumps or measles) or bacterial meningitis. Making a distinction is irrelevant as it does not affect management, and investigation to exclude an acoustic neuroma is usually unnecessary if the presence of the impairment in childhood is clear-cut.

Noise exposure

A noise exposure history should be taken, as asymmetric exposure occurs commonly from gun-fire. Here there are some misconceptions as to which ear is more likely to be exposed. Guns that are fired from the shoulder, such as a rifle, expose the ear nearer the gun barrel. In right-triggered individuals this is the left ear. If there is a definite history of the audiometrically poorer hearing ear having been more exposed to significantly more noise than the other ear, most clinicians would not investigate the patient further unless there were symptoms such as vertigo which are not normally associated with noise trauma.

Head injury

Head injuries are common but many victims do not seek medical advice at the time. Even if

Table 6.1 A 'guesstimate' of the relative incidence of the various aetiological factors considered to be responsible for asymmetric sensorineural thresholds

Aetiology	Percentage
Unknown	85
Vestibular syndromes	10
Acoustic neuroma	4
Congenital and infections	2
Noise	1
Head injury	1
Drugs	1

they do, hearing is often not considered. When a patient gives a history of a head injury, one has to decide in retrospect whether it is responsible for the impairment. This is extremely unlikely unless there was a temporal bone fracture (Browning *et al.*, 1982) and when this has occurred the patient will be fairly definite about a cause/effect relationship. A history of bleeding from the ear or disequilibrium at the time of injury will also make a fracture more likely. When the head injury was minor or not in the region of the temporoparietal bone, then a fracture as the cause of asymmetric thresholds is unlikely.

Drugs

Only one ear is affected in 60 per cent of patients with documented aminoglycoside ototoxicity (Lerner *et al.*, 1983) and this is likely to apply to other drugs as well. The only occasion when one can eliminate the requirement to screen for an acoustic neuroma because of ototoxicity is when there is a definite cause/effect relationship. This is most likely to be reported if the asymmetric loss of hearing occurred during a hospital admission when an aminoglycoside may have been administered or the patient was in renal failure.

Investigations for acoustic neuroma

In the majority of patients there will be no obvious explanation for the sensorineural hearing impairment following the taking of the history. It is difficult to lay down guidelines as to whom to investigate, as this is a situation where clinical judgement is important. Individuals with neurological symptoms or signs must be investigated. Patients who have disequilibrium or a noticeably progressive unilateral hearing impairment should also be investigated. Some would suggest that the presence of unilateral tinnitus, even if there is no asymmetry in the pure tone thresholds, merits investigation. Unfortunately, the prevalence of tinnitus in the general population is high and there is no evidence that individuals with a neuroma are more likely to have tinnitus than individuals who do not have a neuroma. In making a decision, it is also helpful to ask the question: 'If an acoustic neuroma were to be detected, would its surgical removal in this patient be warranted?' In general, acoustic neuromas grow slowly and if one were identified in an elderly patient it could be argued that its removal was not justified as the chances were low that the patient would ever have anything more than a hearing impairment.

Referral patterns to ENT clinics vary and therefore the proportion of patients with a neuroma will vary between clinics. The proportion of patients investigated will also vary depending on many factors. There are some otologists who always appear to be diagnosing a neuroma, whereas there are others that never do. In a routine otological clinic about 2–3 per cent of those screened will have a neuroma. In clinics with a large secondary referral rate the incidence of neuromas may be considerably higher.

Screening options

There is some debate as to how to screen. The two main options are radiology or audiometry. There is no doubt that magnetic resonance imaging (MRI) with contrast has the best sensitivity of all and will detect small intracanalicular tumours which computerized tomography (CT) scanning with contrast will miss. CT scanning with contrast, however, has as high a sensitivity in extracanalicular tumours. Unfortunately there are many clinics where MRI or CT scanning is not readily available and they are always more costly than audiometry. So one possibility is to screen all patients by audiometry and only to carry out MRI or CT scans on those that fail.

Table 6.2 gives the sensitivity and specificity of the various audiometric tests. The only acceptable tests are those with a sensitivity of better than 90 per cent, that is the test will correctly identify at least nine out of ten tumours. This excludes speech, caloric and loudness balance as potential screening tests, and leaves auditory brainstem response (ABR) and acoustic reflexes to consider. Neither of these tests is reliable or practicable if the thresholds in the affected ear are greater than 70 dB HL. This is likely to be the case in 15 per cent of patients being screened (Swan, 1989) and such patients should go straight to CT or MRI. In those able to be tested, virtually all patients with an acoustic neuroma will be detected by ABR (*Table 6.3*) or acoustic reflexes, and the numbers without an acoustic neuroma going on to sophisticated radiology will be reduced by 60 per cent. Thus, of 100 patients with an asymmetric sensorineural hearing impairment being screened by audiometry, of whom five have an acoustic neuroma and 95 do not, the five acoustic neuroma cases will fail ABR or acoustic reflex screening, and of the 95 that do not have an acoustic neuroma 38 will fail. Thus the numbers requiring sophisticated radiology will be reduced from 100 to 43 (5 + 38), that is they are reduced by 57%.

Some suggest combining the results of ABR and acoustic reflexes, there being three ways of doing this: (a) one test has to be positive; (b) both tests have to be positive; or (c) if the first test is positive, carry out the second test to look for two positive results. Unfortunately, the first protocol (a) is no better than one test alone. The second two protocols (b and c) reduce the false-alarm rate by increasing the specificity but unfortunately also reduce the sensitivity (hit rate) to unacceptable levels (see Appendix I).

Radiological screening

Straight X-rays and tomograms to look for widening of the internal auditory meatus have no role to play because of their low sensitivity of 75 per cent. Contrast myelography has been abandoned because of its side-effects in comparison to CT or MRI scanning. Both of these are improved by the use of gadolinium contrast, though this adds to the expense. CT scanning carries the risks of irradiation, particularly to the eyes. Some patients find being in the CT chamber too claustrophobic. MRI is in most centres more expensive (by up to twice) but will diagnose small intracanalicular tumours down to 3 mm with modern techniques. In most centres, the decision between CT and MRI is based on their availability.

Table 6.2 Sensitivity and specificity of audiometric tests in detecting acoustic neuromas

	Sensitivity ('hit rate')	False negative	Specificity	False alarm
Auditory brain stem	95	5	64	36
Acoustic reflex threshold	100	0	37	63
Acoustic reflex decay	91	9	59	41
Alternate binaural loudness balance	84	16	40	60
Calorics	80	20	50	50
Speech	78	22	60	40

Table 6.3 Tumour size by auditory brain stem response sensitivity

Study	Overall sensitivity (%)	Tumour size > 2 cm	< 2 cm	< 1 cm
Chandrasekhar *et al.* (1995)	93	100	90	83
Gordon and Cohen (1995)	88	100	88	69

(After De Michele and Ruth, 1996)

NF2 acoustic neuromas

Intracranial vestibular schwannomas can be genetically inherited by dominant transmission in chromosome 22: neurofibromatosis 2 (NF2). Such patients usually develop neuromas elsewhere intracranially and sometimes meningiomas. This is distinct from the genetic transmission in chromosome 21 of von Recklinghausen's disease (NF1) which gives *café au lait* spots and skin neurofibroma but rarely acoustic neuroma.

The recognition of patients with NF2 is important because management tends to be conservative. Most will usually present with more than one tumour and life expectancy from then on is 15 years with the possibility of developing

further neuromas or meningiomas anywhere within the central nervous system. NF2 should be suspected in anyone developing an acoustic neuroma below 30 years of age as well as those with a family history. Chromosome analysis is indicated to confirm this. MRI scanning of the entire intracranial cavity and spinal cord should then be done to identify silent tumours.

Management is then directed at making life as disability-free as possible until death. Thus, excision of an acoustic neuroma when there is usable hearing has to be balanced against the risk of loss of hearing in the other ear because of the high risk of developing bilateral acoustic neuromas.

Management of acoustic neuromas

Historically, acoustic neuromas were usually diagnosed when they were so large that they presented with symptoms of increased intracranial pressure. Under these circumstances, surgery was essential to save life. Today, because of the availability of CT and MRI, the majority of tumours are diagnosed when small (*Table 6.4*). It is known from temporal bone studies that 0.7 per cent of the population have a small undiagnosed acoustic neuroma at death (Schuknecht, 1974). This would suggest that some tumours are extremely slow to grow in size and that watchful waiting could be a valid management strategy, particularly in the

elderly or unfit. On the other hand, the larger the tumour at the time of surgery, the more dangerous the surgery, and the more likely are complications such as facial palsy. Preservation of hearing is increasingly being discussed as an aim and this is certainly important in patients with NF2. On balance, watchful waiting is more likely to preserve useful hearing than surgery. Several different surgical approaches are available, the choice being primarily made by the type of surgeon that leads the team. Otologists favour a translabyrinthine or a mid-cranial fossae approach and neurosurgeons a retrosigmoid approach.

Table 6.4 Size of acoustic neuromas at diagnosis

| | Intrameatal | 0–10 mm | Extrameatal | | |
			11–25 mm	26–40 mm	> 40 mm
Denmark					
1976–83	0.7	14	26	24	36
1983-90	0.6	21	29	28	22
West of Scotland					
1985–92	5	11	44	29	15

Translabyrinthine approach

The internal auditory canal is opened via the mastoid and after drilling out the semicircular canals and vestibule. This invariably destroys the hearing but in the majority preserves facial nerve function. This approach is seldom traumatic to the brain or brain stem and is preferred for all but large extracanalicular tumours.

Retrosigmoid approach

This gives wide exposure for large tumours but requires the brain stem to be retracted. It has the potential for preserving the cochlear nerve, and thus hopefully the hearing.

Mid-cranial fossae approach

This requires retraction of the cerebrum and a good knowledge of the internal auditory canal anatomy. Theoretically, this approach gives the best possibility of preserving the facial and cochlear nerves in cases of small tumours.

■ Conclusions

- In a clinic population more than a third of individuals will have a difference in their air-conduction thresholds of 20 dB or more and the commonest reason is the presence of a conductive defect in the poorer ear.
- In a clinic population approximately 15 per cent of individuals will have asymmetry in their bone-conduction thresholds once the effect of any conductive defect has been accounted for.
- The majority of individuals in the general population with asymmetric bone-conduction thresholds do not have an acoustic neuroma, the probability being between 1 in 700 and 1 in 1400.
- Noise exposure, ototoxicity and head injuries are considerably commoner aetiologies than acoustic neuromas but even then account for only a small percentage of cases. The diagnosis in these instances is best arrived at by taking the history.
- The aetiology of asymmetric sensorineural thresholds will remain unknown in the majority of individuals.
- Which individuals with asymmetric thresholds should be screened to exclude an acoustic neuroma is primarily a question of clinical judgement.
- In a routine ORL clinic the choice of which test to use as the initial screening test will depend very much on what facilities and expertise are available. Though brain stem elec-

tric responses might appear to be the best single audiometric test, considerable expertise is required to achieve good results. Sophisticated radiology (CT or MRI with contrast) is more sensitive and specific but is more expensive.
- Surgical removal of acoustic neuromas is usually advisable when diagnosed, though observation is a valid strategy in the more elderly with small tumours because growth is sometimes slow.
- A translabyrinthine approach, though destroying the hearing, preserves facial nerve function in most, and post-operative recovery is quicker.
- A retrosigmoid or mid-cranial fossae approach can preserve the hearing.
- NF2 neuromas are genetically inherited, patients usually presenting below the age of 30 years with a single neuroma, but MRI scanning will often detect other intracranial or spinal neuromas which at that stage are silent. A more conservative approach is usually adopted in such patients.

Further reading

De Michele, A.M. and Ruth, R.A. (1996). The diagnostic use of auditory brainstem response and evoked otoacoustic emissions in the era of magnetic resonance imaging. *Current Opinion in Otolaryngology & Head and Neck Surgery*, **4**, 356–359.

Evans, D.G.R. and Ramsden, R.T. (1995). Neurofibromatosis type 2. *Recent Advances in Otolaryngology*, **7**, 181–189.

Swan, I.R.C. and Gatehouse, S. (1991). Clinical and financial audit of diagnostic protocols for lesions of the cerebellopontine angle. *British Medical Journal*, **302**, 701–704.

7 Sudden hearing loss

'Sudden hearing loss' to many equates with a sudden, idiopathic sensorineural loss, forgetting that many truly sudden losses have a definable aetiology, such as wax.

The otologist should be wary about accepting that a hearing impairment came on suddenly without further enquiry. Patients who become aware of their impairment for the first time on a specific occasion do not have a sudden loss but may report it as such. The time over which an impairment has to occur to be a 'sudden' loss has never been defined, but it is generally taken as a few days. In most instances only one ear is affected.

Identifiable aetiologies in external ear

Wax

Getting water in the ear or impacting wax against the tympanic membrane with a cotton bud or ear-mould can cause a sudden loss that is easy to diagnose and remedy.

Identifiable aetiologies in middle ear

Otitis media with effusion

Otitis media with effusion (OME) following an upper respiratory tract infection is common and causes a variable impairment over a few days. Frequently it is bilateral and the patient usually knows to try and clear the ear by performing a Valsalva manoeuvre.

Identifiable aetiologies in the inner ear

Ear surgery

Though it might not be admitted, ear surgery is probably the commonest cause of a sudden, sensorineural hearing loss. A total or partial hearing impairment can follow any ear operation, the risk depending on the surgeon's expertise, the operation being performed and whether a middle ear infection coexists or occurs subsequently. The risk is highest at the time of surgery, especially if the oval window has been opened or if a semicircular canal fistula was present or created, but the loss can also occur any time post-operatively.

In the immediate post-operative period, inner ear damage should be suspected if there is vertigo associated with spontaneous nystagmus. Audiometry is mandatory in such circumstances. The post-operative ritual of performing the Weber test with a tuning fork is impossible to interpret mainly because of its inconsistencies (see p. 12) but also because the patient frequently has a bilateral conductive impairment. Bone-conduction audiometry with masking of the non-test ear is not compromised by the presence of an ear dressing because it is unnecessary to place the vibrator on the mastoid, the temporal region being quite adequate. Air-conduction thresholds are less easy to obtain because of the dressings but they are less relevant to monitor than the bone-conduction thresholds.

Should inner ear damage be suspected, a decision has to be made as to whether the ear should be re-explored. In general, most otologists would initially monitor the patient for several days. Others might re-explore in the hope of sealing off a perilymph leak, especially following a stapedectomy, but the risk of causing further inner ear damage has to be taken into consideration.

Head injury

It is estimated that in the UK there are nearly 1 million attendances at hospital or general practice with a head injury per year and, in a proportion, the auditory system will be affected. The external auditory canal may be filled with blood, as might the middle ear. The tympanic membrane might be ruptured. The ossicular chain may be dislocated. The temporal bone may be fractured. The auditory nerve may be stretched in its canal and the brain stem and cerebrum may be traumatized. The incidence of each has not been ascertained but permanent sensorineural impairments caused by temporal bone fractures are perhaps commoner than realized. This is because standard skull X-rays are not particularly successful in detecting skull base fractures. Correspondingly, an otoscopic examination should be performed in all individuals with a head injury to ensure that temporal bone fractures are not missed. They are usually evident by blood or cerebrospinal fluid (CSF) in the external auditory canal. Five per cent of all minor head injuries with a short period of post-traumatic amnesia (Browning and Swan, 1982) and 25 per cent of all severe head injuries (Browning, unpublished observations) will have otoscopic evidence of a temporal bone fracture and the majority of these will not have been detected on standard X-rays.

Classically, fractures are classified as longitudinal when a blow to the parietal or temporal region creates a fracture which runs along the roof of the external auditory canal, through the middle ear, then anterior to the cochlea to the region of the carotid artery. This is the commonest type of fracture and seldom causes more than a conductive impairment. Transverse fractures are less common but are much more likely to injure neurological structures. These result from a severe blow to the front or back of the head causing a skull base fracture with multiple fracture lines which can go through various parts of the cochleovestibular system and temporal bone.

The subdivision of temporal bone fractures into longitudinal and transverse fractures is a clinical rather than pathological one. Pathological studies have conclusively shown that in a temporal bone fracture there are usually multiple fracture lines with an extremely variable pattern (Travis et al., 1977). This has been confirmed clinically now that CT scans are more frequently used. Once a fracture is detected the problem is one of management. If a conductive hearing impairment is present, the patient should be reviewed 6 months later. By this time any blood in the ear will have been absorbed and any tympanic membrane tear will have healed. If a conductive impairment is still present, then it is likely to be due to ossicular chain dislocation which can often be surgically corrected. Any sensorineural impairment, as shown by poorer bone-conduction thresholds on the side of the fracture, is most probably due to a perilymph leak through the fracture site rather than due to stretching of or direct damage to the auditory nerve. As the majority will settle spontaneously, a wait and see policy is adopted. Exploration is only indicated to seal off a continuing CSF leak but to do so adequately could entail both a middle cranial fossa and a mastoid approach to ensure the site was detected.

Rarely is the facial nerve damaged sufficiently by a fracture to result in a palsy. Convention has it that if this is immediate in onset the mastoid should be explored and the site of trauma to the facial nerve identified. It is rare for it to be completely transected but removal of bone spicules and alignment of any traumatized segments is considered beneficial.

Individuals who do not have a temporal bone fracture are unlikely to have damaged the peripheral auditory system, but a considerable proportion will have central auditory problems (Gatehouse 1983) and disequilibrium due to whiplash injuries to the brain stem (Fischer *et al.*, 1997).

Blast injuries

A rarer variant of a head injury is a blast injury to the ear, commonly these days from an explosion in civil disorders. Another common cause is a slap on the ear with the open palm of the hand. These usually result in a tear of the tympanic membrane, but a sensorineural impairment can also result.

Barotrauma (round window rupture)

Rupture of the round window membrane can occur due to barotrauma after an aeroplane flight or after underwater swimming or diving. How this can occur is worth explaining.

The external auditory canal, middle ear and inner ear are three individual compartments, separated by the tympanic and the round window membranes, respectively (*Figure 7.1*). The pressure in the external auditory canal is that of the environment. The pressure in the middle ear is that of the environment, unless the Eustachian tube is malfunctioning. The pressure in the inner ear is also that of the environment, except when transiently increased by any action which raises the intracranial pressure such as coughing or sneezing. This is then transmitted from the CSF to the inner ear via the cochlear aqueduct. A pressure difference between any two of the three compartments can cause the intervening membrane to tear.

During aeroplane ascent, the atmospheric pressure and hence that of the external auditory canal and inner ear can fall to around 540 mmHg. This equates to about 10 000 feet high in a non-pressurized aircraft and to the pressure usually maintained in a commercial aircraft (Farmer and Gillespie, 1997) (*Figure 7.2*). Even if the Eustachian tube is functioning poorly, the excess middle ear air can escape down the Eustachian tube so that the pressure difference between the middle ear and the other two compartments readily equalizes. During an aeroplane ascent it is thus uncommon to have otalgia due to a differential pressure across the tympanic membrane. The main problem arises during descent, when the pressure in the external auditory canal and inner ear returns to normal. The middle ear is then at a lower pressure with respect to the external auditory canal and the inner ear (*Figure 7.3*). Even a normally functioning Eusta-

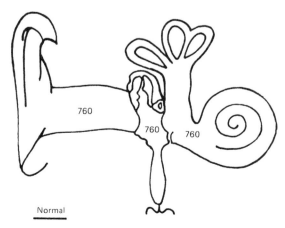

760

760   760

Normal

Figure 7.1 Normal pressures in the outer, middle and inner ears (mmHg)

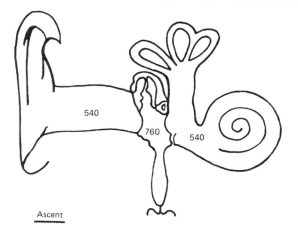

Figure 7.2 Typical pressures during aeroplane ascent (mmHg)

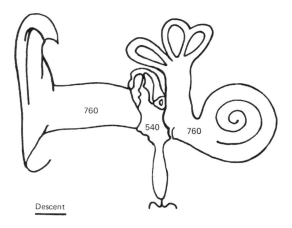

Figure 7.3 Typical pressures during aeroplane descent (mmHg)

chian tube can fail to open against this pressure differential and more so if the tube is oedematous because of an upper respiratory tract infection. So otalgia is common during an aeroplane descent and on occasions the tympanic membrane can rupture. Alternatively, the round window membrane may rupture and perilymph can leak into the middle ear. This is considered more likely to occur if there is an additional increase in inner ear pressure occasioned by a cough or a sneeze, but this only increases the pressure by ~ 1.5 mmHg.

Similar pressure differentials occur during subaqua diving. Thirty feet (10 metres) underwater is equivalent to an additional 1 atmosphere (760 mmHg) of pressure. However,

most divers perform a Valsalva manoeuvre regularly and effectively.

Deep sea divers are another group to consider because there are several reasons why such individuals might have hearing problems after a dive. Otitis media with effusion can occur due to rebound vasodilatation of the middle ear and Eustachian tube mucosa, but is not too difficult to diagnose. Rupture of the tympanic membrane should also present little diagnostic difficulties. What can sometimes be difficult to differentiate between is decompression sickness and barotrauma causing a round window rupture. Decompression sickness is often associated with disequilibrium but there should be no nystagmus.

In individuals with a sudden sensorineural hearing loss recent aeroplane flights and diving should be enquired about. If the round window has ruptured, vertigo and nystagmus will almost invariably be present and if this is not the case then the diagnosis must be doubted. Reports of round window ruptures following coughing, sneezing or straining must be treated sceptically considering that the round window membrane is a closely knit fibrous structure (Normura *et al.*, 1983) and coughing, sneezing or straining only raises the intracranial pressure by 1.5 mmHg (150 mmH$_2$O).

Having made a diagnosis of round window rupture, what next? The majority will heal spontaneously and efforts to encourage this by avoiding increases in intracranial pressure are warranted. Bed rest with the head elevated and the avoidance of coughing, sneezing and straining at stool are suggested. Monitoring of the patient's hearing is often easiest when the patient is in hospital, though hospitalization is by no means necessary. The majority stabilize rapidly within 10 days without surgical intervention. However, if at any time the severity of the vestibular symptoms increases or the bone-conduction thresholds continue to decrease, then exploration of the middle ear may be warranted. The surgical techniques are well described elsewhere but for the less experienced it is worth stating that the round window membrane cannot be seen in the round window niche via a posterior tympanotomy (*Figure 7.4*). It can be visualized only by drilling away the overhanging bone of the promontory. Almost certainly some reports of 'round window ruptures' are due to misinter-

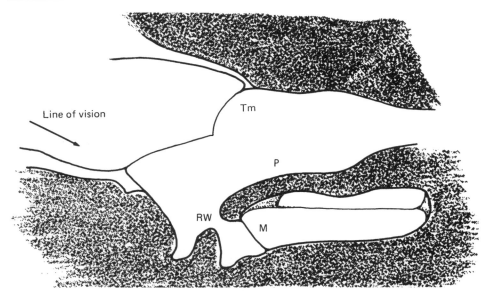

Figure 7.4 Transverse section of the ear showing that direct visualization of the round window membrane (M) in the round window niche (RW) is not usually possible via an anterior tympanotomy. P = promontory; Tm = tympanic membrane

preting the frequently present circular holes in the mucosal folds in the niche as 'tears'. True tears of the membrane are linear and often extremely difficult to visualize (Normura *et al.*, 1983).

Drugs (Table 7.1)

The drugs most likely to cause a sudden as opposed to a progressive hearing loss are the aminoglycosides. In developed countries their use is primarily restricted to those in hospital. The exception to this is ear drops (see below). Audiometric monitoring of those on systemic aminoglycosides has its supporters, but there is the practical problem of doing this in patients who are frequently extremely ill and unable to perform pure tone audiometry. Aminoglycosides are usually also vestibulotoxic so the development of vertigo is frequently the first clinical symptom. If concern is raised the antibiotic should be changed as some degree of recovery in hearing frequently occurs. Fortunately, more careful prescribing of aminoglycosides with monitoring of serum levels, especially in those with renal failure, has led to a fall in the incidence of cochleovestibular side-effects. Cisplatinum antimitotic therapy can also

cause a truly sudden hearing loss, but patients on such therapy are readily identifiable.

Many take salicylates for various ailments but the development of tinnitus is a warning sign. Fortunately, salicylate ototoxicity is self-resolving once the drug is stopped.

The evidence to support beta-blockers and loop duretics being ototoxic is less strong, particularly in patients with normal renal function. Of course, it is not just the drug that could be responsible for a hearing impairment but the condition for which the drug is being taken, such as cardiovascular disease, could also be implicated.

Ear drops

Ear drops may be indicated in otitis externa and active mucosal chronic otitis media. Frequently they contain an aminoglycoside (*Table 7.2*) and where there is potential direct contact of the drops with the round window membrane, and perhaps the oval window, there is the potential risk of ototoxic damage both to hearing and balance. That such damage can certainly occur in laboratory animals is not doubted, but reported cases in humans with chronic otitis media are few. Studies that have monitored the hearing prospectively during

Table 7.1 Commonly prescribed cochleotoxic drugs

Class	Drug	Property names
Non-steroidal anti-inflammatory	Salicylates	Alka-Seltzer Antoin, Benoral, Claradin, Codis, Hypon, Labofrin, Levius, Unadox, Paynocil, Sofapryn, Veganin
Beta-blockers	Propranolol	Angilol, Apsolol, Bekolol, Inderal
	Acebutolol	Sectral
	Atenolol	Tenormin
	Labitolol hydrochloride	Trandate
	Metoprolol tartrate	Betaloc, Loprisor
	Nadalol	Corgard
	Oxprenolol hydrochloride	Apsolox, Trasicor
	Pendolol	Visken
	Sotalol hydrochloride	Beta-Cardone, Sotacor
	Timolol maleate	Betin, Blocadren
Antibiotics	Gentamicin	Cidomycin, Garamycin Genticin
	Amikacin	Amikin
	Framycetin sulphate	Soframycin
	Kanamycin	Kannasyn, Kantrex
	Neomycin	Mycifradin, Nivemycin
	Netilmicin	Netillin
	Tobramycin	Nebcin
Loop diuretics	Frusemide	Dryptal, Frusetic Frusid, Lasix
	Bumetanide	Burinex
	Ethacrynic acid	Edecrin
Metals	Cisplatinum	Neoplatin

Table 7.2 Antibiotics in commonly prescribed topical eardrops, often in combination with topical steroids

Antibiotic	Preparation
Clioquinol	Locortin-Vioform
Framycetin	Sofradex
Gentamicin	Cidomycin Genticin Gentisone HC
Neomicin	Audicort Betnesol N Neo-Cortef Otomize Predsol N Tri-Adcortyl Otic Vista-Methasone N
Neomycin and polymyxin	Otosporin

treatment of active chronic otitis media with potentially ototoxic ear drops are also few. One study that did so in 88 patients detected no change in thresholds (Browning *et al.*, 1988). Unfortunately, this does not mean that it cannot occur, albeit rarely. As with aminoglycosides given systemically, the development of vertigo or imbalance is an important warningxx symptom and the drops should be stopped.

Syphilis

Very rarely, early acquired syphilis is complicated by meningitis and this usually presents with various neurological symptoms and signs. The auditory nerve may be involved and there are reports of deafness being the sole presenting symptom. Because it is important to treat syphilitic meningitis there is an argument for routinely performing syphilis serology in individuals with a sudden sensorineural hearing impairment.

Acoustic neuroma

In about 10 per cent of patients with an acoustic neuroma, the hearing impairment is reported to have come on suddenly. This does not mean that they were seen immediately following the loss nor that the loss was truly sudden. It could be that the patient just happened to notice the loss on a specific occasion. Because of the relative rarity of acoustic neuromas it would be incorrect to imply that an individual with a sudden hearing loss is likely to have one. However, it would seem prudent to consider screening individuals with a unilateral sudden loss for an acoustic neuroma in the same way that one would do for an asymmetrical sensorineural impairment (see p. 61).

Idiopathic sudden sensorineural hearing losses

Despite the taking of a full history and performing a clinical examination, many individuals will have none of the causes of a sudden hearing loss discussed above. The aetiology is thus a matter of conjecture, viral infections and vascular events being the most favoured reasons.

It is often suggested that if a patient has had a recent upper respiratory tract infection, then a viral infection is responsible. Unfortunately at any one time one-third of the population will have, or will recently have had, such an infection. So even in the presence of a raised viral antibody titre, the relationship with a sudden hearing loss must be doubted.

Vascular events could occur because of some abnormality in the blood or blood vessels. There is some evidence to support altered filterability of red cells or blood and plasma viscosity (Hall *et al.*, 1991; Ciuffetti *et al.*, 1991; Ohinata *et al.*, 1994). There is little histological evidence to support pathological vascular abnormalities, though arterial spasm could occur. With the advent of MRI the aetiology may become clearer in the next decade.

What investigations, if any, should be done in this idiopathic group? Acoustic neuroma and syphilis are probably the only diagnoses that are necessary to exclude, though many would perform several other investigations.

Whether any audiological investigations need to be done in the acute stage, apart from pure tone audiometry, is doubtful.

Management

Many different forms of management have been proposed. These are summarized in *Table 7.3* and are discussed more fully in other texts (Booth, 1997). Their very multiplicity implies that none is of proven efficacy. They mainly have the objective of increasing the blood flow through the cochlea. Steroids in theory could minimize damage irrespective of the aetiology. Most forms of medical treatment have reported ~ 60 per cent 'resolution' rate and this is likely to reflect the natural, untreated 'resolution' rate. Until a controlled trial of the management has been reported, all forms of

Table 7.3 Drugs prescribed for idiopathic sudden hearing impairments

Class	Examples
Vasodilators	Nicotinic acid, betahistidine, hyoscine, atropine, inhaled carbogen
Anticoagulants	Heparin, phenindione
Lowering blood viscosity	Low molecular weight dextran
Steroids	ACTH, prednisolone
Vitamins	Lipoflavinoid

medication should be considered unproven and unlikely to be superior to doing nothing. Medication is not without its side-effects, occasional deaths having been reported, especially from intravenous therapy.

What is suggested is that no therapy should be given to those with an idiopathic loss, and the hearing impairment be allowed to recover spontaneously. This approach may appear nihilistic but it is, in practice, what most otologists do as the majority no longer make any real attempt to have patients with a sudden hearing loss referred to them. This is probably an incorrect attitude as there will certainly be a small number where there is a definite form of management. It is necessary to see all individuals with a sudden hearing impairment in order to identify this small portion but the vast majority will require no specific therapy and will recover spontaneously.

■ Conclusions

• Hearing impairments that come on suddenly are relatively uncommon.
• They have to be distinguished from hearing impairments that are noticed for the first time on a specific occasion.
• The minority are idiopathic in origin and the otologist should first ensure that one of the recognized aetiologies is not responsible.
• Wax, otitis media with effusion and ear surgery should be easy to identify.
• Active surgical intervention may be needed on the rare occasion that a fistula, following barotrauma or a temporal bone fracture, does not heal spontaneously.
• The initial diagnosis of a temporal bone fracture is by otoscopy rather than by conventional skull X-rays. CT scans are more helpful but are not always available initially.
• A round window rupture is only likely to follow a definite change in atmospheric pressure such as occurs following an aeroplane flight or underwater diving. It is also unlikely to have occurred unless there is vertigo as well as a hearing impairment.
• Drug ototoxicity should always be considered and, if there is doubt, any drug the patient is on should be stopped and an alternative prescription given.

• Though it is extremely unlikely in the absence of other neurological signs, syphilis should be excluded by serological tests as therapy is important to institute.
• Once the above causes have been excluded, the condition must be considered idiopathic.
• The majority of sudden hearing losses are idiopathic and at present there is no proven form of medical or surgical management for them. Thankfully the majority recover spontaneously.

Further reading

Booth, J.B. (1997). Sudden and fluctuated sensorineural hearing. In *Otology*, Vol. 3, Chap. 17, Scott-Brown's Otolaryngology, 6th Edition. Butterworth-Heinemann, Oxford.

Farmer, J.C. and Gillespie, C.A. (1997). Pathophysiology of the ear and nasal sinuses in flight and diving. In *Basic Sciences*, Vol. 1, Chap. 7, Scott-Brown's Otolaryngology, 6th Edition. Butterworth-Heinemann, Oxford.

Fischer, A.J.B.M., Verhagen, W.I.M. and Huygen, P.L.M. (1997). Whiplash injury. A clinical review with emphasis on neuro-otological aspects. *Review of Clinical Otolaryngology*, **22**, 192–201.

8 Exaggerated thresholds and non-organic hearing loss

In a routine clinic, exaggerated thresholds are uncommon because the patients are motivated to respond. On the other hand, when individuals are claiming for noise-induced deafness, they are likely to exaggerate their impairment to some extent. A different situation to be aware of is where a patient appears to be attention-seeking because of their hearing impairment. Such individuals, if of normal hearing, sometimes feign a unilateral impairment and, if bilaterally impaired, a more marked impairment than they truly have.

In all cases, the otologist's aim is to recognize that the thresholds are being exaggerated and to ascertain what are the true thresholds.

Clinical assessment

Clinicians are unlikely to identify exaggerated thresholds unless they are suspicious. They should be particularly wary if the patient exaggeratedly strains to hear what is being said, this being atypical even in the profoundly impaired. Being alerted, the next task is to confirm exaggerated thresholds without the patient realizing that they are being assessed. If the patient has a hearing aid, the first task is to remove it on some pretence such as 'Can I see what type of aid you have?'. Conversation then carries on about general matters, the clinician's aim being to assess whether speech-reading is necessary for comprehension. Speech-reading is not possible when the clinician is writing in the case notes or examining the ear. In patients with a severe impairment, speech-reading is vital. Most otologists have their own particular tricks. Some make apparently harmless conversation in a quiet voice when doing something else, such as examining the ear. When doing this, questions in a quiet voice such as 'Am I hurting you?' will often be responded to.

Free-field voice testing can also be helpful. The patient's responses are often slower than normal, presumably with the aim of implying that it is difficult. The responses can sometimes be a deliberate mistake, for example 'cowgirl' being replied instead of 'cowboy'.

If a unilateral impairment is claimed, a Stenger tuning fork test can be performed (see Appendix VI). It might seem a counsel of perfection to suggest that this should be performed routinely when a patient has a unilateral impairment, even if exaggerated thresholds are not suspected. On the other hand, frequently performing the test gives practice in interpreting the responses.

Audiometric assessment

Pure tone audiometry

If a non-organic loss is suspected prior to audiometry, it is important to ask the person testing the patient to look for signs of exaggerated responses. More importantly, the patient should be carefully instructed how to respond. It is relatively easy to exaggerate thresholds by simply altering the technique of response from 'when *you think* you can hear the tone' to 'when *you can definitely* hear the tone'. This increases the thresholds by 10–15 dB. Another technique is to respond at each frequency at a level that sounds equally loud above one's true threshold.

The manner and in particular the speed at which a patient responds may be slower than normal because they want to indicate that it is difficult. The method of response can also be helpful, especially if they have been asked to raise a finger when they hear the tone, rather than press a button. The delightful name of 'malinger-finger' describes well the initial flicker of a finger which occurs soon after a tone has been presented, which is then rapidly suppressed.

If a patient is responding faithfully, the thresholds are usually determined over a narrow range of sound levels. For example if a patient's real threshold is 20 dB HL, signals 10 dB above this threshold at 30 dB HL will almost invariably be heard. In exaggerated losses the range over which the threshold is determined is often considerably wider. The main exception to this is the elderly who often find it difficult to make up their minds. It is also normal for a patient to make a few false-positive responses when no signal has been presented. This does not occur when the loss is being exaggerated and until this occurs the thresholds are likely to be artificially elevated.

It is unfortunate that thorough pure tone testing takes time, patience and experience.

If a unilateral or grossly asymmetrical impairment is being claimed it is important to assess the bone-conduction thresholds in each ear without masking. Normally, when assessing bone-conduction thresholds, the transcranial attenuation is taken as 0 dB but in many circumstances it can be higher (*Table 8.1*). However, 25 dB is the level at which it would almost invariably occur at 0.5 and 1 kHz, so that even when testing the bone conduction in a dead ear, a sound 25 dB above the bone-conduction threshold of the better ear should be heard. If a patient does not report hearing a tone in the poorer hearing ear 25 dB above the bone-conduction threshold in the better ear, then a non-organic loss is likely. This is provided the patient has been instructed to report when they hear a sound, irrespective of where they hear it. Individuals who are exaggerating their loss are often unwilling to admit to hearing a sound when it is presented to their claimed poorer hearing ear.

In testing the air conduction thresholds, the median level of transcranial attenuation of air conduction is ~ 60 dB (*Table 8.1*). If, without masking, there is a difference in the proffered air-conduction thresholds of 60 dB or greater, then exaggerated thresholds should be suspected. Exaggerated thresholds cannot be proven, however, until the thresholds are asymmetric by 80 dB or more.

Results

When noise-induced loss is being claimed the shape of the audiogram can indicate exaggerated thresholds. It is not necessary to have a notch in the audiogram in patients with noise trauma but in sensorineural impairments the

Table 8.1 Transcranial attenuation

		Mean	0.5 kHz	1 kHz	2 kHz	4 kHz
Air conduction	Minimum	41	45	40	40	40
	Maximum	79	75	75	80	85
	Median	60	55	60	60	65
Bone conduction	Minimum	−6	−10	−5	−5	−5
	Maximum	31	25	25	35	40
	Median	10	10	5	10	15

(After Snyder, 1973)

higher frequencies are usually more severely affected than the lower. The audiogram should thus be sloping rather than flat. It might be expected that the exaggerated audiogram would mirror the true thresholds but this is not always the case because recruitment at the higher frequencies makes sounds above the threshold sound louder than they really are. A flat rather than a sloping audiogram should make one suspicious of exaggerated thresholds (*Figure 8.1*).

In many instances when the thresholds are exaggerated, there is an artificial air–bone gap, brought about by the fact that it is more difficult to exaggerate bone- than air-conduc-

tion thresholds. False air–bone gaps in individuals claiming noise-induced hearing loss confuse the issue as it is generally agreed that the bone conduction is used to assess inner ear function. A Rinne tuning fork test, if negative, is an indicator of a conductive defect (see p. 10).

If exaggerated thresholds are suspected the audiogram should be repeated after telling the patient that the results are not as accurate as they might be and reinstructing them in how to respond. This gives them the opportunity to respond more accurately without any embarrassment, as well as correcting any real misunderstanding there may have been. The

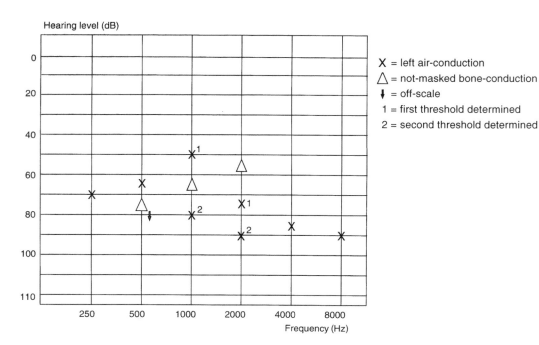

X = left air-conduction
△ = not-masked bone-conduction
↓ = off-scale
1 = first threshold determined
2 = second threshold determined

Figure 8.1 Typical audiogram in non-organic hearing loss

amount that a loss is exaggerated is often no more than 10–20 dB but this can make a considerable difference to the amount of compensation paid.

It is easy to suggest that, if unreliable thresholds are elicited, pure tone audiometry should be abandoned and reliance placed on slow vertex electric response audiometry (ERA). This attitude does not take into account the inaccuracies of ERA (*Table 8.2*), so it is worth persevering and attempting to get accurate thresholds by pure tone audiometry. The other considerable disadvantage of ERA is that it assesses the air-conduction thresholds. When there is a true conductive component to a hearing impairment, the bone-conduction thresholds are used for compensation purposes. Unless electrocochleography is resorted to the only way bone-conduction thresholds can be assessed is by pure tone audiometry.

Audiometric Stenger test

In the presence of asymmetric thresholds, the audiometric Stenger test can be used to gain a reasonable estimate of the real difference between the ears (see Appendix VI).

Acoustic reflexes

In patients being assessed for compensation, some would suggest that tympanometry and

Table 8.2 Correlation between pure tone and slow vertex thresholds at single frequencies in organic losses

| Within (dB) | Percentage | |
	Series A[*]	Series B[*]
0	32	29
5	60	46
10	72	62
15	80	73
20	86	82
25	92	90
30	94	94
35	96	96
40	98	97
45	100	98

[*]Series A after Davis (1984) and series B after Coles and Mason (1984)

acoustic reflex tests should be carried out before pure tone audiometry. It is not that the results themselves are important but the patient is given the impression that this is a test which cannot be fooled. As such, the test should be performed in a manner which enhances its image as a 'lie detector'. It is then hoped that the patient will try harder during pure tone audiometry.

The sound level at which an acoustic reflex is elicited can be a pointer to exaggerated thresholds. In those with normal hearing, the reflex thresholds will be at least 60 dB greater than the pure tone threshold. In those with a sensorineural impairment the difference will be less because of recruitment. Even then there is usually at least a 20 dB difference between the reflex and the pure tone thresholds. If the thresholds are within 20 dB, a non-organic element to the loss is likely. If the reflex threshold is lower than the pure tone threshold at any frequency, then a non-organic element is certain.

If there is an apparent air–bone gap (see above) it would be helpful if its presence be confirmed and an absent acoustic reflex *may* be helpful in doing this (see p. 41).

Speech audiometry

Speech audiometry can be of particular value in detecting exaggerated thresholds. The reason for this is that patients often find it more difficult to exaggerate the impairment in speech as opposed to pure tone audiometry. The task in speech audiometry is to repeat the words and there is less chance that the instructions will be misinterpreted.

It is important to note the words repeated back because the mistakes made can be informative. Normally mistakes are primarily made with the consonants rather than the entire word.

The half peak level elevation (HPLE) (see p. 193) should be compared with the average of the two best pure tone thresholds. Normally the results are within 15 dB. In individuals exaggerating their impairment the difference is often considerably larger, the HPLE on the speech being better than expected.

Electric response audiometry (ERA)

Many consider ERA to be an objective test but this is not the case if inexperienced observers interpret the results. To aid such individuals and to eliminate bias, more rigid protocols for performing and analysing the results are often used. Slow vertex (cortical) responses are more frequently used than brain stem responses as they are often specific, but they can be considerably different (*Table 8.2*) from those obtained by pure tone audiometry (Davis, 1984; Coles and Mason, 1984). For practical purposes the difference should be considered to be as much as ±15 dB (90 per cent confidence limits) though on occasions there will be individuals in whom the discrepancy is as much as 25 dB.

The accuracy of ERA improves considerably when the results at two or more frequencies are averaged and compared with the pure tone thresholds. Considerably fewer data are available to calculate how much this improves the accuracy but Coles and Mason (1984) reported that when three or more frequencies measured from slow vertex ERA are averaged and compared with the pure tone average at these frequencies, the overlap (95 per cent confidence) between the mean thresholds is 9.5 dB, the ERA giving the better thresholds.

Electrocochleography is seldom necessary, as adults are usually co-operative in allowing ERA to be performed. The exception to this is when it is important to assess the bone-conduction thresholds.

■ Conclusions

• It is important to suspect exaggerated thresholds in individuals who have been exposed to significant amounts of noise.
• Patients who are likely to gain psychosocial support for having a hearing impairment are also likely to exaggerate their thresholds.
• The otologist is usually the first to suspect exaggerated thresholds, mainly by noting inconsistencies in the patient's ability to hear.
• When suspected, the results of pure tone audiometry, speech audiometry and acoustic impedance can be compared to identify discrepancies.
• The audiometric Stenger test can be used in individuals with an asymmetric impairment to give an estimation of the true difference between the ears.
• Once exaggerated thresholds have been suspected, the aim is to assess the true

thresholds. If time is taken these can usually be obtained by pure tone and speech audiometry.
• The threshold obtained by slow vertex evoked response audiometry at a single frequency should be interpreted with caution. Averaging the thresholds over at least three frequencies gives considerably greater accuracy.

Further reading

Alberti, P.W. (1981). Non-organic hearing loss in adults. In *Audiology and Audiological Medicine*. Edited by H.A. Beagley. Oxford University Press, New York, pp. 910–931.
Coles, R.R.A. (1982). Non-organic hearing loss. In *Otology*. Edited by A.G. Gibb and M.F.W. Smith. Butterworths, London, pp. 150–176.

9 Hearing aid provision

The process of hearing aid provision

The provision of a hearing aid is a multistage process that in many cases involves more than one provider. *Table 9.1* lists the various stages in the usual order in which they are carried out along with who might do so at each stage. At most stages there are several possible providers, the choice being dependent on what staff are available and the degree of subspecialization within a department.

Who sees the patient first varies from country to country but there is usually a choice of two routes open to the patient and their family. There is the medical one, and this is appropriate if there is concern about the ears medically. This route is also an initial requirement in most countries that provide aids as part of the health care system. Having passed the medical as-sessment (see below) the patient can then be provided with an aid within or outside the health care system from a hearing aid dealer. The alternative is to purchase an aid directly from a hearing aid dealer and hope that he will be bound by the ethical and trading rules of his profession. This includes the requirement that patients do not fail certain criteria which necessitate a medical opinion (Swan and Browning, 1994).

In the UK, the primary care physician (GP) often has the option of bypassing the medical (otolaryngological) opinion and referring directly to an audiology department for the fitting of an aid. Such 'direct referral' schemes are not available everywhere and patients going via this route still need to be screened

Table 9.1 Stages in hearing aid provision as most commonly practised

Stages	Medic	Aud Sc	Professional involved Tech	HT	Com
Candidature	✔	✔	✔		✔
Medical assessment	✔				
Audiometric assessment		✔	✔		✔
Choice of ear/s	✔	✔	✔		✔
Choice of aid	✔	✔	✔		✔
Aid fitting		✔	✔		✔
Rehabilitation		✔	✔	✔	✔
Benefit assessment		✔	✔		

Medic = medical personnel; Aud Sc = audiological scientist or audiologist; Tech = audiometric technician; HT = hearing therapist; Com = commercial personnel

as to whether they fail any medical criteria. If such criteria are strictly adhered to, up to 50 per cent of patients seen by a private hearing aid dispenser or in a 'direct referral clinic' are likely to fail one or several of the criteria (Swan and Browning, 1994).

Medical assessment

The medical consultation, which is usually provided by an otolaryngologist, has four different objectives:

- To identify otological symptoms in addition to a hearing impairment, such as tinnitus, ear discharge and vertigo, which might merit investigation and management other than with a hearing aid.
- To identify ear pathology such as active chronic otitis media that may merit investigation and management because it is a disease. This is usually done by otoscopy.
- To identify, by a combination of otoscopy, clinical tests of hearing and audiometry, ears with a conductive impairment which could benefit from surgery to improve the hearing.
- To identify, by a combination of the history, clinical tests of hearing and audiometry, patients with an asymmetric sensorineural impairment who may merit investigation to exclude an acoustic neuroma.

Thereafter, it is decided whether the patient is likely to be a suitable candidate to benefit from an aid. If this is the case the degree that the otolaryngologist is involved thereafter depends on their interest and whether they have a supervisory role with respect to the service.

Candidature: who is likely to benefit from an aid?

The answer to this question is anyone with a hearing impairment confirmed by audiometry and who is motivated to try one. So, if a patient is willing to try an aid they should be provided with one for a trial period. Though the above is the case the median threshold of individuals seeking advice about amplification is 45 dB HL (Lancet Editorial, 1987) which suggests that patients do not consult until they are moderately disabled. The proportion of the impaired population that possesses an aid is surprisingly low (*Table 9.2*). Thus only 55 per cent of those with an impairment in their better ear of between 55 and 65 dB HL have an aid. There are several interrelated reasons why this is the case: not wanting to appear disabled; belief that aids do not really help; acceptance of poorer hearing with age; a lifestyle that does not demand good hearing; and in some the perceived cost. This is not to say that aids will not benefit those with lesser impairments; 10 per cent of aids are currently being issued to those with pure tone averages less than 30 dB. This proportion is likely to increase with the development of aids that do not amplify at the low frequencies as these are frequently normal in the early stages of a sensorineural impairment (*Figure 9.1*).

It is commonly felt that 'the majority of aids end up in a drawer'. This may have been the case with body aids but with appropriate fitting, adequate follow-up and instruction in the use of an aid, 95 per cent of individuals issued with a behind-the-ear aid report use and benefit from it (GRI clinic data).

Table 9.2 Possession of a hearing aid as a function of the degree of hearing impairment in the better hearing ear

Degree of impairment dB HL	% possessing aid	% of aid owners
< 25	< 1	7
25–34	10	8
35–44	30	18
45–54	35	21
55–64	55	18
65+	90	28

(After Davis, 1997)

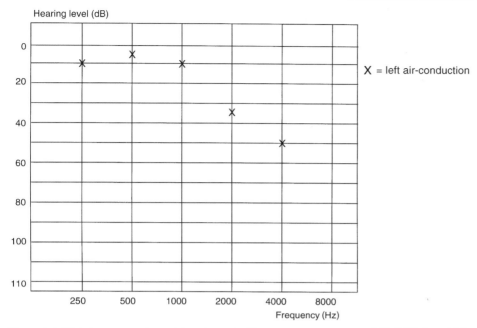

Figure 9.1 High tone sensorineural impairment with a pure tone average of 25 dB HL for which provision of an aid is practical and beneficial with modern aids

Choice of ear/s: monaural or binaural fitting

It would seem appropriate in a patient with a bilateral hearing impairment to attempt to fit two, rather than one, aid. However, this is seldom achieved for several interrelated reasons. The first is the cost. The second is wearer resistance to the concept. 'I'm not so bad as to require *two* hearing aids, am I?' is a common reaction. Thirdly, the majority of hearing aid users are over the age of 65 and as such their physical ability to cope with small, technical aids is limited, though it is not nearly as bad as some would suggest. Fourthly, the added benefit of the second aid is small in comparison to the first. Finally, aids can be uncomfortable to wear, often giving a blocked-up sensation and can in some situations make listening worse by amplifying unwanted background noise.

On the other hand, individuals who have previously been satisfactorily aided monaurally frequently return stating that their aid is of less value than it used to be. This is most frequently because their hearing has deteriorated and often the thresholds are poorer than 70 dB HL. In such cases the first thing to consider is a more powerful aid with a well-fitting mould but the concept of wearing binaural aids is usually readily accepted by these patients as they have little to lose and a considerable amount to gain. The unaided ear will be making no contribution to the hearing but, if bilaterally aided, central summation of input from two ears can in effect improve the loudness by around 6 dB. Most patients in this group will try binaural aids and 80 per cent will continue to use them both (Day *et al.*, 1988). Those that do not usually have an asymmetric impairment with one considerably poorer ear.

However, it should never be forgotten that binaural aids are a possible option in anybody being fitted with an aid. The fact that a patient has an asymmetric impairment should not exclude them from being considered for binaural aids. Theoretically it is almost impossible to provide them with balanced hearing but a monaural aid does not give balanced hearing either.

Monaural fitting: which ear?

For all these reasons the majority of first aid issues are likely to be monaural rather than binaural. The question then arises as to which ear to fit and, in arriving at a decision, there are various factors to consider, the most important being whether the patient has symmetric or asymmetric hearing. An individual is usually considered to have asymmetric hearing if the pure tone thresholds in the ears are different by 10 dB or more averaged over the frequencies 0.5, 1, 2 and 4 kHz. In an average ORL clinic there are likely to be one symmetric for every three asymmetric impairments (GRI clinic data), the commonest reason being a super-added conductive component in one ear.

Asymmetric hearing

The rule to apply is: 'Fit the poorer hearing ear unless the thresholds are poorer than 70 dB HL, when the better ear should be fitted'. The rationale for this is as follows. When the hearing thresholds are poorer than 70 dB HL aids are technically more difficult to fit because they need a well-fitting mould to prevent feedback, gains may be insufficient and distortion can be a problem. If the hearing is better than 70 dB HL in both ears then patients expect to get the aid in their poorer ear and in a cross-over study of side of use (Swan et al., 1983) 92 per cent reported greater benefit with an aid in their poorer ear. Why should this be when individuals achieve higher speech discrimination scores for speech from in front when they are wearing the aid in their better hearing ear? The easiest answer is that their main disability is when the speaker is on their poorer hearing side and an aid in their poorer hearing ear is of considerable benefit to them in these circumstances. If they were to wear the aid in their better ear, they would not hear the speaker any clearer and the aid could introduce unwanted background noise, making it more difficult than it would have been without the aid. An additional reason is that many aid wearers turn it off when they do not need to hear or when there is background noise. If the aid is in their poorer ear they will be minimally worse off when it is switched off. They would be worse off if the aid was in their better ear.

Symmetric hearing

In individuals with symmetric pure tone thresholds there are no acoustical reasons for choosing one ear rather than the other. In these circumstances the decision as to which ear to fit would logically be dictated by other factors but in the many instances it is uncertain as to how these will influence the final choice of side (see below). If a behind-the-ear (BTE) aid is being provided one option is to manufacture two moulds and let the patient decide.

Specific requirement reasons

The majority of individuals do not have a specific requirement to hear better on one side than the other but a British taxi driver might wish to wear it in his left ear in order to hear the passengers better. Such reasons are not common and the major requirement to consider is which ear is used on the telephone. Most hearing-impaired individuals have minimal trouble hearing on the telephone partly for the reason that over 80 per cent of them (GRI clinic data) use their better hearing ear on the phone. In such cases a BTE aid in their better ear would be a nuisance rather than a benefit. In those with an in-the-ear (ITE) aid it could be a benefit.

Practical reasons

In deciding which side to fit, manipulative difficulties due to a stroke or joint problem are often said to be an important reason for choosing a side. However, it is often difficult to predict the side in which the patient will find it easier to manipulate the aid. It is by no means certain, for example, that the right ear is the correct ear to put an aid in when the right hand is dominant. There are several different ways of inserting and manipulating an aid and, providing it can be done, any method is 'correct'. So manipulative difficulties are a case for issuing bilateral moulds and letting the patient try both sides. Manipulative reasons often dictate the type of aid that should be provided. Body aids have the largest controls. BTE aids can be more difficult to position than ITE aids but the controls in these are smaller.

Pathological reasons

It is the accepted rather than the proven rule that it is undesirable to fit an aid to an ear with chronic otitis media, the concept being that it will encourage the condition to be active. If possible, then, aids are fitted to an ear with an intact tympanic membrane but this can mean fitting it to the better hearing ear. Frequently there is bilateral disease, so if surgery can create an intact tympanic membrane and perhaps improve the hearing some would suggest this should be the initial management. Sometimes it is impossible to avoid fitting an ear with active or inactive chronic otitis media because the patient does not want an operation, because the operation fails or because the individual has bilateral disease. Under these circumstances patients often find it valuable to have bilateral moulds so that they can vary the side they wear the aid in, depending on which side is discharging. A vented ear mould is often suggested as being helpful in these circumstances but there is no evidence that this is so.

Audiometry in hearing aid fitting

Pure tone audiometry

The air-conduction thresholds are required to choose the most appropriate gain and frequency response of a hearing aid for a particular ear. How these are used will be discussed later.

Loudness discomfort levels/uncomfortable loudness levels

These are the frequency-specific pure tone loudness levels at which a patient reports that the sound is 'uncomfortably loud'. These levels can be recorded on a standard audiogram chart (*Figure 9.2*). From this the dynamic

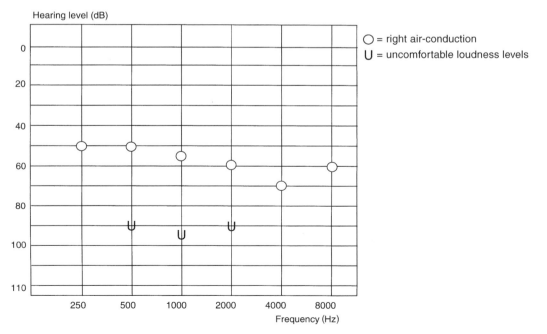

Figure 9.2 Loudness discomfort levels recorded as an audiogram. In this case the dynamic range is small, the discomfort levels (U) being less than in a normal hearing individual because of recruitment

range between being able to hear a tone (i.e. the threshold) and it becoming uncomfortable can be measured. In a normal hearing individual the dynamic range is 90–100 dB. In individuals with a hearing impairment this is reduced not only because of the raised thresholds but in some by recruitment. Hence the common complaint by the hearing impaired: 'Don't shout, I'm not deaf'. This limited dynamic range can give problems with hearing aid fitting.

Speech audiometry

Some centres recommend speech audiometry to exclude ears with poor optimal discrimination scores from candidature for aid provision. A more practical use is to measure benefit (see below).

Which aid and mould?

Physiological considerations

Though the majority of humans have not retained the ability to move their pinnae, it is still of considerable value to them as it acts as a collecting horn with a baffle system of cartilaginous folds which directs sounds into the external auditory canal. That it is beneficial is exemplified by the habit of cupping the hand behind the ear to enlarge its size in order to hear better. The pinna and the external auditory canal both have an effect on the frequency spectrum of sound which finally arrives at the tympanic membrane (*Figure 9.3*), but the contribution the pinna makes to this is a minor one

and is dependent on the angle from which the signal comes in relation to the head.

The pinna also contributes to sound localization, the brain being able to interpret minuscule variations in sound pressure levels and timing of the sounds arriving at the ear or ears. Only one ear is actually necessary to localize sound, as the necessary variations in sound pressure level can be achieved by minor head movements which change the relative position of the pinna and the ear to the sound. Localization in the horizontal plane is helped by the use of two ears, primarily because of the addition of the head shadow effect and the different times of arrival of the sound at the two ears.

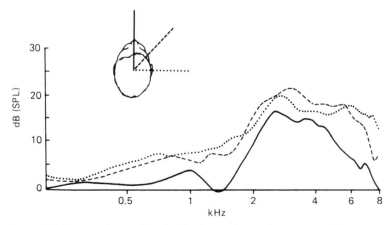

Figure 9.3 Increase in sound level at the tympanic membrane caused by resonance of the external auditory canal and the baffle system of the pinna. The effect of different angles of sound incidence is shown by the different lines (after Weiner and Ross, 1946).

Localization in the vertical plane is a function of the degree to which high frequency tones (∼ 7 kHz) are reflected by the pinna.

The wearing of a behind-the-ear or body aid obviously alters the method of transmission of sound from the environment to the middle ear, as the sound collecting mechanism of the pinna is not utilized. As the microphone of in-the-ear aids is in the external auditory meatus these aids theoretically are likely to be superior to other aids in sound localization. In practice they are not for two main reasons. Firstly, the concha is filled up by the aid and secondly, the effects of the pinna are mainly at the higher frequencies which are not amplified by present-day aids. Completely in-the-canal aids where the microphone is in the canal can potentially utilize the effect of the pinna at the frequencies it amplifies.

All aids have an ear mould and this inevitably has an acoustical effect as it blocks and shortens the ear canal which will modify the resonance frequency of the ear (*Figure 9.4*).

Aid models

Aids that amplify air-conducted sounds can be worn on the body, behind-the-ear (BTE), in-the-ear (ITE) or completely in the canal but they are all similar in that they have a microphone to receive the sound which is then amplified and delivered to the ear. The smaller the battery size, the less power they contain and the more quickly they are used up. Because of the close position of the microphone to the ear canal, ITE and completely-in-the-canal (CIC) aids tend to feed back at lower gains than BTE aids and are usually only suitable for those with a mild to moderate hearing impairment. The smaller the aid the less space there is for electronic modification. For example, not all ITE aids have a telecoil. This lack of space can be overcome to some extent by having a remote control keypad.

Because of common perceptions most patients would prefer to have an ITE aid because it is considered to be less noticeable. This

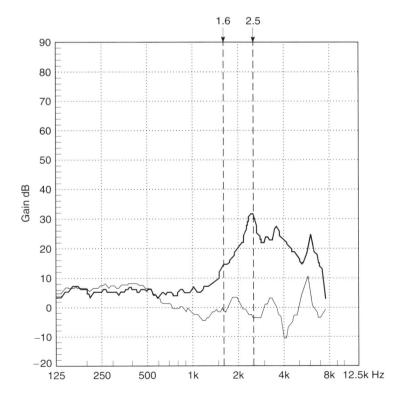

Figure 9.4 Insertion gain of a normal open ear canal (top graph) which is eliminated by wearing an ear mould (lower graph)

perhaps is only really the case in those with short hair. Because the aid is within the mould some find it easier to insert than a BTE aid. Though the volume control is smaller some find its position easier than that on BTE aids and it usually incorporates the on/off switch. Sometimes the small size of the canal precludes the use of a CIC aid.

Aids that transmit sound via bone conduction and cochlear implants that convert sound to electrical energy are discussed elsewhere (see pp. 104 and 124).

Acoustical data

Manufacturers provide certain acoustical data for each aid which have been measured on artificial ears (couplers). These are average results and are not the same as those achieved in real ears because of the varying effect of the ear canal anatomy in different patients (see below). However coupler data on gain, frequency response and maximal output are used for the initial choice of an aid.

Gain
An aid has to be able to amplify sound sufficiently for it to be heard at a level that improves the hearing but is not so loud that it is uncomfortable. The acoustical gain of an aid is represented as a frequency response curve (*Figure 9.5*) when the aid is set at maximal gain on the volume control with an input sound pressure level at the level of speech, usually 60 dB SPL.

Frequency response
This is ascertainable from the gain chart. In addition the frequency response of most aids can be varied to different degrees by a screw (or screws) to give low or high frequency emphasis (*Figure 9.5*). Some aids have a greater range of modifications available than others. It is also possible to have a remote control that changes the frequency response for different listening situations.

Maximal output
This is a similar response curve but with an input sound level of 90 dB SPL (*Figure 9.6*).

Other characteristics

Many different options are available, some giving added using options (e.g. telecoil, audio input), others being acoustical.

Telecoil
Most aids have a telecoil (T) position on the switch that turns the aid off (O)/or the microphone on (M). Sometimes there is also an 'MT' (microphone and telecoil on) position. The 'T' position isolates the aid from environmental sounds so that it can pick up sound by electromagnetic induction from telephones and television or in public meeting places (cinema, theatre etc.) that have been fitted with loops. An aid at the 'T' position thus excludes unwanted background noise and increases the signal-to-noise ratio.

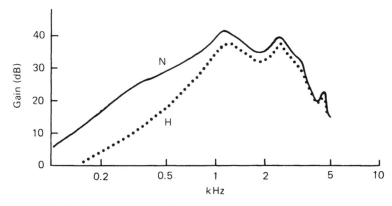

Figure 9.5 Gain characteristics of an aid represented as a frequency response curve. On this graph, the frequency response of two different settings are shown. N = normal tone setting; H = high tone setting

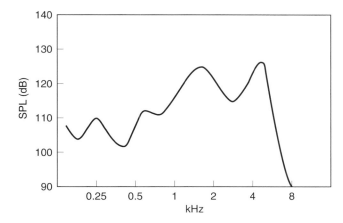

Figure 9.6 Maximal output of an aid, represented as a frequency response curve

Audio input

The output from a radio or personal compact disc player can be fed directly via an electric cord to a socket on the aid.

Automatic gain control

When an aid is set towards its maximal gain, two things can happen which could disturb the wearer. Speech varies in volume and, as such, peak clipping of the louder elements could occur with subsequent distortion of the speech. Unexpected loud noises could also be uncomfortable for those with recruitment. Automatic gain control, often achieved by compression, hopefully overcomes these problems.

Microphone

Most microphones are omnidirectional but vary in their position depending on the type of aid. They are usually above the pinna in BTE aids, in the concha in ITE aids and in the canal in CIC aids. In theory ITE and ITC aids can utilize the acoustical effect of the pinna at the frequencies they can amplify. Directional microphones enhance the pick-up of sounds in a particular direction and can improve the signal-to-noise ratio.

Adaptive response

Some aids are programmed to automatically adjust the gain at different frequencies depending on the signal's characteristics. The term 'automatic signal processing' is sometimes applied to such aids.

Ear moulds

With ITE and CIC aids the acoustic mechanism is housed within the mould. In general they are tailor-made for an ear and cannot be reused in the other ear or in other patients. This is in contrast to BTE aids which only need a different mould to do this. Modular ITE aids overcome this to some extent, as the ear mould is a housing for a removable mechanical part.

The looser a mould is the more comfortable it is to wear, mainly because the ear feels less blocked. It also removes the occlusion effect which makes the patient's voice sound louder because of the conductive loss a tight mould gives. The problem with loose moulds is feedback. An alternative is to drill a small (≤ 1 mm) vent hole in the canal piece (*Figure 9.7*) which is unlikely to cause feedback and has a negligible acoustic effect (see below). Venting can also be done on ITE aids and some would argue that it should be routine in all mild and moderate hearing impairments.

With BTE (and body) aids there is a considerable variety of modifications that can be made to an ear mould, the choice being dictated by a number of factors. Confusion can arise because of uncertainty about the names of various parts of the mould. To overcome this the internationally accepted nomenclature should be used (*Figure 9.8*).

Style

In order to make moulds less obvious and more comfortable to wear, a mould for a BTE

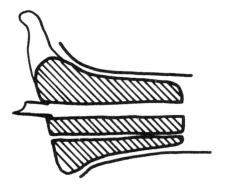

Figure 9.7 Non-acoustic 1 mm vented mould to relieve blocked-up feeling

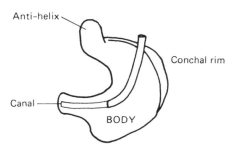

Figure 9.8 Different parts of ear moulds for BTE aids

aid can be skeletonized to different extents (*Figure 9.9*).

Material

Moulds are usually made of hard acrylic but when a tight-fitting mould is required in a severe/profound impairment the canal piece or the entire mould can be made of soft acrylic. For the extremely rare patient who is truly allergic to acrylic a silicone mould can be made. Irritant reactions to materials used to disinfect/clean the mould (bleach, washing-up

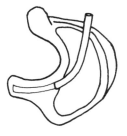

Figure 9.9 Skeleton mould

liquid, TCP etc.) are a commoner problem which, if enquired about, should be easy to identify.

Acoustic modifications

Venting with a 2 mm vent can decrease the low frequency gain of a hearing aid complex (*Figure 9.10*) but can only be used with a mild to moderate impairment because of feedback. The canal length can be varied; the shorter it is the larger the remaining volume of the canal, which results in a peak in the sound pressure around 2 kHz.

Connecting tubing and elbow

In BTE aids there is a choice of diameter and configuration of the connections to the ear mould. A large internal diameter tube enhances the high frequencies. The elbow can also be used to enhance the high (e.g. Libby horn) or the low frequencies. A filter can be inserted in the elbow or tubing to flatten out peaks in the response.

Fitting strategy

Usually the first decision is the style of aid which depends on availability (ITC and CIC aids are not available routinely in British NHS practice), patient requests, special listening requirements and cost. ITC and CIC aids are usually ruled out for those with a severe or profound impairment because of feedback. The next consideration is the degree of impairment taken from the air-conduction thresholds which will determine the gain required. Several rules are available to calculate this, but the easiest is the half-gain rule which is based on the finding that patients with a sensorineural impairment do not want speech amplified as much above their threshold of sound detection as a normal individual does. Thus a normal patient with 0 dB HL thresholds wishes to hear speech at around 60 dB SPL. A hearing-impaired patient with 40 dB HL thresholds does not wish to amplify speech to 100 dB SPL. Experience has shown the required figure to be at half the impairment level, in this instance $40 \div 2 = 20$, that is a gain of 20 dB, which would give the individual amplified speech at $60 + 20 = 80$ dB SPL.

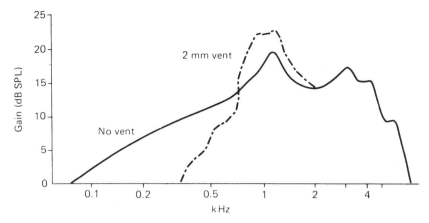

Figure 9.10 Acoustic gain of a hearing aid complex with a 2 mm parallel vented mould compared to the same complex with a non-vented mould

The next aspect to consider is the frequency response. Several different prescription routes are possible.

Try and hope it is beneficial

In the past, and still today in many centres, the policy was choose what was thought to be the best aid and mould, make some adjustments if there was a sloping sensorineural impairment and issue the aid. This was a very reasonable strategy to adopt when there was only a limited range of aids, such as former British NHS aids, available. There is no doubt that the main determinant for aid use is careful instruction as to how to insert the mould, position the aid and adjust the controls. If this is done (see below) up to 95 per cent of individuals will report using their aids. However, this does not mean that they achieve optimal benefit and that acoustical modifications would not improve upon this.

Try different acoustical settings

When BTE aids are being considered it is easy once a mould has been made to try different aids and different acoustical settings. The patient is then asked which they prefer. An alternative is to carry out free-field aided audiometry (see p. 91) and see which aid they score best with. There are many problems with this approach; the aid that initially sounds the best does not necessarily give the best performance and with time individuals learn

and adapt to their aid so that aided scores at fitting are not those achievable 6 months later.

Match frequency response to audiogram

Several different prescription strategies have been advocated which take into account the gain required at each frequency, the loudness discomfort levels and whether it is a conductive or sensorineural impairment (e.g. Byrne and Dillon, 1986). When initially formulated these strategies were calculated from the audiogram and the aid characteristics measured in a $2 \, cm^3$ coupler. Now they are used with real ear insertion gains (see p. 90).

Measure frequency response in comparison to audiogram

The availability of equipment to measure in a specific patient the actual sound level arriving at the tympanic membrane has to all intents and purposes outdated the other methods of prescription. There is an argument that such measures ought to be carried out routinely as only 40 per cent of aid complexes have an appropriate acoustical output if the fitter just looks at the audiogram and makes what they think are the appropriate adjustments (Swan and Gatehouse, 1995). Unfortunately it is not possible to predict which audiograms are difficult to fit. For example a 'ski slope' sensorineural loss is no more difficult than a high tone sensorineural loss.

Though the real ear gain can be made to

come within certain prescription targets (Natural Acoustics Laboratory (NAL), see Byrne and Dillon, 1986) most centres just 'eyeball' the graph to see if it fits rather than doing any calculations. If calculations are to be done then calculation of the speech intelligibility index is probably a better option (see p. 91).

Audiometry in hearing aid evaluation

Real ear insertion gains

The patient is sat with their aid inserted, in a quiet non-reverberant room in front of two loudspeakers set at 45 degrees on either side of the mid-line. A small bore tube is inserted past the ear mould into the ear canal towards the tympanic membrane. The hearing aid is then set to a comfortable listening level. Pure tone sound is then presented sweeping over the range 0.25–8 kHz and the level of the amplified sound arriving at the tympanic membrane is displayed on a monitor (*Figure 9.11*). The advantage of this type of measurement over coupler (i.e. artificial ear) measurements is that the acoustical properties of a patient's ear canal along with those of the mould are taken into account. The patient's

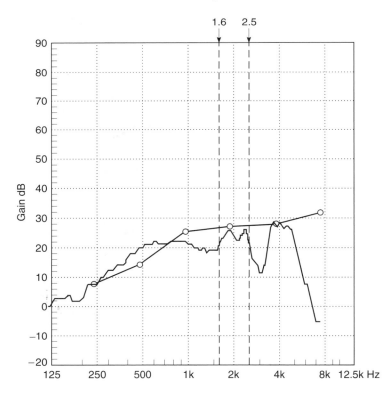

Figure 9.11 Insertion gains. The line connecting the circles is the NAL based gain required in this patient at different frequencies based on the pure tone thresholds. The other line is the real-ear-insertion gain in this patient with an aid, adjusted to try and achieve the ideal NAL gain. In this instance it does so but the frequency response is irregular and an attempt at smoothing should be made using filters

pure tone thresholds are also displayed so that modifications to the frequency response of the hearing aid complex can be made to ensure that sound is sufficiently amplified over the full frequency spectrum. This can be done by 'eyeballing' or by using a mathematical model (e.g. NAL Byrne and Dillon, 1986).

Aided thresholds

This can be done for pure tone thresholds or speech. The patient is seated in a similar position as for insertion gains. The patient's thresholds/speech reception are measured, first unaided and then with a hearing aid/aids set at the most comfortable listening level.

Speech intelligibility index

Some components of speech are more necessary for speech comprehension than others. This particularly applies to the higher frequencies especially when speech-reading is not possible. The speech intelligibility index (SII) is the proportion of a normal speech signal that is available for a person to hear. This is calculated using a software program from the patient's pure tone thresholds and the insertion gain measurements (*Figure 9.12*). Different aids and adjustments can be made to give an optimum SII.

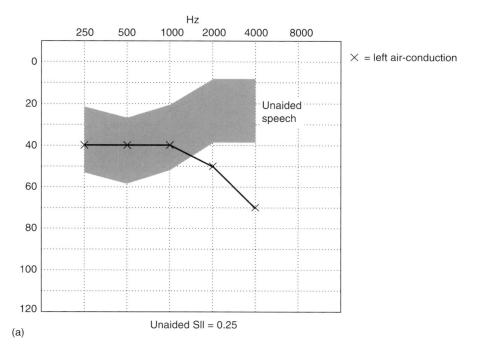

(a)

Figure 9.12 Speech intelligibility index. (a) The air-conduction thresholds in the left ear are plotted as normal. The shaded area represents the frequency and loudness spectrum of normal speech at 65 dB. This patient can hear that proportion of speech in the shaded area that falls below the pure tone thresholds. This percentage of the total shaded area is the patient's speech intelligibility index (SII) and in this case is 0.25 or 25%.

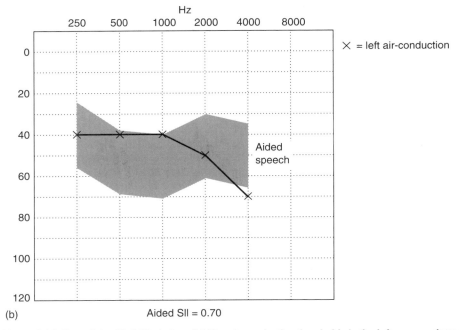

(b)   Aided SII = 0.70

Figure 9.12 Speech intelligibility index. (b) The air-conduction thresholds in the left ear are plotted as before. In this case the speech has been amplified by a hearing aid whose gain and frequency output known and which results in the shaded area of speech shown on the graph. The percentage of this that can now be heard has increased, giving a speech intelligibility index of 0.70, i.e. 70 per cent. The speech area can be varied by inserting into the computer program different hearing aid characteristics to maximize the speed intelligibility index

What follow-up?

It is a common attitude that individuals who have been provided with a hearing aid will come back if they have any problems. Several studies have shown that this is not the case. First, some patients do not realize that they are having difficulties as exemplified by the number of times that patients are seen who consider that their ear mould is properly in but the anti-helix is sticking out (*Figure 9.13*). Second, patients often attribute a lack of benefit to the hearing aid rather than to themselves; there are people who think that hearing aids always whistle! Finally, patients are often embarrassed about troubling the hospital staff because 'they are busy'. Though they might be busy, the time spent on examining, testing and providing a hearing aid is totally wasted if an aid is not worn. It does not take long to assess whether a patient has acquired the necessary skills to use his aid and to correct any problems there may be. Follow-up of all patients issued with a hearing aid is thus extremely important.

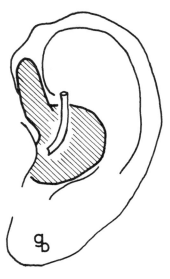

Figure 9.13 Incorrect insertion of ear mould, in part due to large anti-helix of the mould which can be removed to ease insertion

Table 9.3 is a list of tasks that an individual should demonstrate they are able to perform, along with the percentage who cannot perform them satisfactorily at the first return visit. One of the easiest ways of running a follow-up clinic is to take the patient through the task list and assess whether they can perform them or not. The order in which the tasks are tested does not matter, the order in the table being a logical one if the patient starts off with the aid in their ear. Any difficulties the patient might have are then easily identified and corrected by further instruction and practice in front of the trainer.

Using a mirror usually does not help. More than a third of patients have difficulty inserting the mould correctly and it is usually because they cannot get the anti-helix in behind the fold of the ear (*Figure 9.13*). It is not uncommon for this to cause ulceration of the underlying skin and of course the gain that can be used is limited because of feedback due to poor fitting. Insertion difficulties can usually be corrected by further instruction, but if difficulty is still encountered there is no good reason, in many patients, to have an anti-helix on the mould. It can be removed by buffing with a disc which makes the mould easier to insert but means it is still held firmly in place by the conchal rim. It is only when a high-powered aid is being used that a tight-fitting ear mould is desirable. There will be a small proportion who will not manage to insert the mould even

Table 9.3 Task list that patients should be asked to carry out at return visits, with the percentage that fail to perform the task at the first return visit after 4 weeks of aid use

Task list	% unable to perform
Remove aid	3
Switch off	25
Change batteries	12
Insert mould	30
Position aid	20
Switch on	25
Adjust volume	25

(GRI clinic data)

when the anti-helix has been removed and for them a small acrylic knob added to the mould can be of benefit.

In the majority of individuals the practical difficulties can be overcome at this return visit, but it is worthwhile bringing those that cannot perform the tasks back for a further visit. If on this occasion they require further instruction they should return until they can perform the tasks satisfactorily. If such a follow-up protocol is practised, 50 per cent of patients will be discharged able to perform the tasks after the first return visit, and 85 per cent after the second visit. In the end 95 per cent of patients report that they are aid users which amply demonstrates the value of a structured follow-up. How much each of them uses the aid will vary and this will depend on their disability and their hearing requirements.

What rehabilitation?

There is no doubt that all patients should be followed up to ensure that they have mastered the skills required to use a hearing aid. What is less proven is the role of speech-reading and auditory training. Part of the difficulty in assessing these things is an inability to measure benefit in that benefit from the use of an aid does not equate with the number of hours the aid is used each day. The amount an aid is used will depend on how often the patient considers they require amplification. An obvious example is that the amount of television

that is watched varies considerably between individuals as does the frequency with which they hold a conversation. So an individual who wears his aid for 1 hour a day to talk to his neighbour but does not watch television may be getting as much benefit from his aid as someone who wears it most of the day to watch the television because the neighbours complain. Another important fact is that the wearing of an aid does not invariably mean that the wearer is benefiting. The most obvious examples are patients who wear their aids and report benefit despite the fact that the batteries are flat. There is certainly an argument that after technically satisfactory aid-fitting the patient should be questioned regarding residual disability, particularly in the circumstances where they are most disabled. This can either be done by questionnaire, (Gatehouse, 1998) or in an open interview. The advantage of the former is that the questionnaire can be completed at home where there is more time to consider the replies. Attention can then be directed at trying to overcome any residual disabilities by counselling concerning tactics, by providing a second aid or by accessory aids.

Accessory listening devices

A hearing aid will be issued to most individuals with an impairment to help them with speech comprehension. However, many do not wear the aid all the time and use it only for certain listening situations such as watching the television. At other times they may still have difficulties such as hearing the doorbell or the telephone ring. So for them assistive listening devices should be considered after the aid has been provided and any residual disabilities identified by interview.

Alerting devices

Loud bells for the door and telephone are available but just as important to consider is their position. A bell sited on the door or in the hall is more difficult to hear than one in the room where most time is spent. It could be moved or an additional bell added. For the severely or profoundly impaired, bells can be complemented by substituting flashing lights. Vibrating devices in alarm clocks can be put under the pillow to wake the patient in the morning.

Telephone amplification

ITE and CIC aids can be used on their own with a telephone, but this is less practical with a BTE aid. Perhaps the best telephone device for use without any aid is one where the volume of the incoming speech can be adjusted within the handset. Some phones have built-in telecoils and can be used with an aid as discussed below. Telecoils are not infrequently built into public telephones and are identified by the symbol of an ear with a diagonal line through it.

Telecoil systems

Most hearing aids have a telecoil (see p. 86) built into them which can be accessed by switching to the 'T' or 'MT' position. Sound is then picked up by electromagnetic induction from a loop system installed in a public room such as a church, cinema or theatre. The speaker's voice is picked up by a microphone and can be more selectively heard against background noise via the loop. Alternatively a telecoil can be built into a telephone and the hearing part of the handset held over the aid.

Television amplification

Many hours are often spent watching the television and if the volume is increased by the hearing impaired this can cause considerable annoyance to others in the house or to neighbours. A hearing aid is not always ideal because it amplifies background noise and what is required is a method of increasing the signal-to-noise ratio. A headset plugged into the television is a good option but mobility is limited by this. A telecoil from the television can be led to the viewer's chair and used with their hearing aid. Finally there is teletext.

Monitoring the service

When they refer a patient for a hearing aid, otolaryngologists will understandably hope that the most appropriate aid/s are provided and that the patient's hearing disability is alleviated by them and perhaps accessory aids. Those in charge of a department will wish to audit the service provided and purchasers may wish to have this information to direct them as to where to spend their money.

Audit requires that there be gold standards with which to compare a service. Unfortunately in hearing aid provision the outcomes used tend to be deficient in recording residual disability. Surrogates such as percentage of patients that use their aid and hours of use are not particularly helpful because wearing an aid does not mean that the disability has been reduced or that a different aid would not be better. Unfortunately audiometric measures of benefit are not routinely used, nor would a single test ever suffice because of the multiple different listening situations there are. It could be that the speech intelligibility index will become a standard basic measure.

Perhaps the best way to evaluate a patient is to enquire as to whether they have any residual disability using any aiding systems they might have. At present it is not possible to overcome all problems and return the patient to 'normal', especially in speech-in-noise situations. However, experience will usually tell you what can and cannot be achieved in a patient with certain audiometric characteristics. Hopefully in the future data will be available, as they now are for cochlear implants, which will give standards which should be achievable in various subgroups of patients.

■ Conclusions

• The provision of a hearing aid is a multistage process with a variety of different providers who can be responsible at each stage.
• In order that the patient gains maximum benefit from an aid it is essential that someone is responsible for monitoring the service.
• Candidature should include anyone with a hearing impairment that is motivated to use a hearing aid.
• The current level of uptake of aids by the hearing impaired is low because of a desire not to be disabled, belief that aids do not really help, the acceptance of the impairment with age, a lifestyle that does not demand good hearing and in some instances cost.
• Medical screening is required to manage other symptoms such as vertigo, to detect pathology such as chronic otitis media and acoustic neuroma, and to offer alternative management for conductive impairments.
• If bilaterally impaired, bilateral aids should be considered. Monaural aids are often preferred because of a patient's attitude and cost.

• Bilateral aids are particularly beneficial in the severely impaired.
• Air-conduction pure tone thresholds are required to choose the gain and frequency response of an aid.
• Behind-the-ear, in-the-ear and completely-in-the-canal aids are appropriate for those with a mild to moderate impairment. The choice is determined by a patient's attitudes, acoustic requirements, specific requirements and cost. Behind-the-ear aids are required for those with a severe impairment because of feedback problems with in-the-ear and completely-in-the-canal aids.
• The ability to measure real ear insertion gains along with a greater ability to alter the frequency response of aids has materially improved our ability to tailor aids for a specific patient.
• Follow-up is essential to ensure that a patient can technically use their aid and to identify any residual hearing disability.
• Accessory listening devices should be considered for any residual disability.

Further reading

Gatehouse, S. (1997). Hearing aids. In *Audiology*, Vol. 2, Scott-Brown's Otolaryngology, 6th Edition. Butterworth-Heinemann, Oxford.

Tyler, R.S. and Shum, D.J. (1995). *Assistive Devices for Persons with Hearing Impairment*. Allyn and Bacon, Boston.

10 Specific management of external and middle ear conditions

General aims

In adults there are usually several reasons for managing external and middle ear conditions. Even if asymptomatic, the condition itself may merit treatment to prevent complications. An example of this is active chronic otitis media where the symptoms can be minimal but complications such as a conductive hearing impairment are likely if the ear goes untreated. However in most conditions the majority of complications are not serious and the main object is usually to relieve symptoms which can be any combination of hearing impairment, ear discharge, ear discomfort or fullness, tinnitus and vertigo. Though such symptoms may be present, the resulting disability can be minor and in some patients not meritous of management.

For ease of presentation, this chapter initially deals with specific conditions, what the potential outcomes are, what investigations are indi-

cated, and how the patient may be managed medically and surgically. Surgery to improve the hearing is almost always an option to consider. To do the latter requires knowledge of the surgeon's own technical results for the type of surgery being proposed. It also requires the patient's disability to be rated and the potential benefit estimated. Because the majority of external and middle ear conditions result in a hearing impairment a section is devoted to bone-conduction aids and in particular to bone-anchored hearing aids (BAHAs). All these aspects are addressed in this chapter. The management with a conventional hearing aid is essentially the same as for a sensori-neural impairment (see Chapter 9). Tinnitus and vertigo are dealt with in Chapters 14 and 15. Otitis media with effusion in children is dealt with in Chapter 13.

Otitis externa

Outcomes

Disease complications

These are uncommon but include stenosis of the canal and malignant otitis externa. The

latter is only likely in immunocompromised patients such as those with uncontrolled diabetes.

Symptoms

The majority have an itchy ear discomfort associated with a mild hearing impairment. The latter is usually due to a combination of canal oedema, retained debris and inflammation of the pars tensa.

Investigation

In the majority no aetiology is identifiable. The history should identify trauma from poking the ear with cotton buds, matchsticks, paper clips etc., or an irritant reaction from cleansing agents such as hair shampoos, antiseptics on ear moulds and ear drops such as Cerumol. Clinical examination should identify associated dermatological conditions such as psoriasis and seborrhoeic dermatitis of the scalp and face. Bacteriological culture is usually irrelevant as the majority of bacteria isolated are normal skin commensals or secondary colonisers as a result of topical antibiotics. Secondary fungal infection is usually recognized otoscopically. Culture is advisable in the uncommon situation where systemic antibiotics are to be given because of spreading cellulitis. Skin-patch allergy testing may be helpful if the condition does not settle and topical antibiotic preparations have been used. Radiology is only necessary in malignant otitis externa.

Management

Surgical

Aural toilet is the mainstay of management, either by syringing by non-specialists or suction by specialists. In the majority of patients this is usually all that is necessary. Unfortunately, toilet is frequently omitted and medication alone supplied.

Medical

Topical or systemic antibiotics are usually unnecessary and can be harmful by causing secondary colonisation with bacteria and fungi as well as causing a topical allergic reaction. Topical steroids (betamethasone 0.1 per cent) relieve the ear discomfort and can be administered by ear drops or by filling the canal with ointment. Sometimes the canal is narrowed by oedema which makes aural toilet difficult. This can be lessened by topical steroids administered on wicks, either gauze or commercial (e.g. Pope wicks). Aluminium acetate or glycerol and icthamol are alternative preparations that can be considered.

Inactive chronic otitis media

Outcomes

Disease complications

Inactive chronic otitis media may become active but the chances of this occurring are not known. There are those that suggest getting the ear wet increases the chances, but the evidence for this is anecdotal. Equally the evidence for the mould of a hearing aid encouraging activity is anecdotal.

Symptoms

Hearing impairment, with or without tinnitus, is usually the sole symptom if the ear remains inactive.

Investigation

Audiometry with appropriate masking will assess the degree of impairment and the magnitude of the air–bone gap in each ear. Otoscopy will assess the size of the pars tensa defect and in many instances the intactness or otherwise of the ossicular chain. The otoscopic findings can then be correlated with the magnitude of the air–bone gap which goes some way to assessing the likely surgical procedures that would be necessary to improve the hearing (see p. 45). The disability resulting from the hearing impairment can be surmised by questioning and by inference from the air-conduction thresholds in both ears (see p. 105).

Management

Non-surgical

Some would give advice about keeping the ear dry to prevent activity. A hearing aid is an option to lessen the hearing disability.

Surgical

A myringoplasty can be performed with the object of creating an intact tympanic membrane, which lessens the risk of future activity. During this procedure, if the ossicular chain is found to be normal, a myringoplasty should also improve the hearing. If the chain is disrupted or fixed and if surgery has the additional aim of improving the hearing then an ossiculoplasty can be performed in addition, the combined operation being called a tympanoplasty.

Healed chronic otitis media

In healed chronic otitis media, activity is unlikely unless the cause of the initial otitis media recurs (e.g. acute otitis media). Hence, the discussion for healed chronic otitis media is the same as that for the hearing aspects of inactive chronic otitis media.

Active chronic otitis media

Outcomes

Disease complications

Active chronic otitis media starts with a pars tensa perforation or a retraction in the attic or middle ear which progressively erodes the ossicular chain, thus increasing the magnitude of the conductive impairment. The air–bone gap is not invariably 60 dB, the maximum possible air–bone gap (see p. 43), because of the differing degrees of adhesion that can occur between the remnants of the ossicular chain and the tympanic membrane. The activity occasionally causes labyrinthitis with vestibular symptoms and/or a sensorineural hearing impairment. On rare occasions intracranial complications can occur (Table 10.1). All these complications can occur with active mucosal disease as well as with cholesteatoma, no one type being 'safe'.

Symptoms

In addition to the hearing impairment (with or without tinnitus) that goes with inactive chronic otitis media an active ear may or may not be associated with an ear discharge.

Investigation

As in inactive chronic otitis media, this involves investigation of the hearing and in addition of the disability caused by the discharge, if any. The correlation between otoscopic activity and patient report of a discharge is low. There are

Table 10.1 Complications of chronic otitis media

Intracranial	n	% cholest.	% non-cholest.
Meningitis	22	41	59
Brain abscess	93	64	36
Subdural empyema	36	69	31
Extradural empyema	19	58	42
Lat sinus thrombosis	36	53	47
Total	150	59	41
Extracranial	n	cholest.	non-cholest.
Post-auricular abscess	65	49	51
Facial palsy	14	14	86
Petrous apicitis	2	0	100
Bezold's abscess	5	0	100
Total	87	41	59

(From Singh and Maharaj, 1993)

Table 10.3 Percentage of the variance in health status accounted for by questions in an ear discharge inventory

Factors	Variance (%)
Mopping and smell	21
Visibility of discharge	15
Frequency of discharge	Not significant

(After Browning, 1997b)

two reasons why this might be the case. The first is that in 20 per cent of active ears the volume of mucopus is insufficient to discharge via the external auditory meatus (Browning, 1997). The second is that the patients are not being asked the correct questions. Some patients feel that their ear runs but cannot support this by evidence such as crusting in the ear, a discharge on the pillow or wet cotton buds (*Table 10.2*). Such more detailed questions should be asked. An even more relevant question to ask is about the smell and their degree of concern regarding this, as this is the aspect that mainly determines their disability (*Table 10.3*). In determining the disability, the frequency of the discharge does not appear to matter in relation to these other factors.

Otoscopy after any necessary suction toilet will classify the type and site of activity (see p. 38). Otoscopy is unfortunately a poor pre-dictor of the likelihood that the activity will be symptomatic because of a discharge, there being agreement in only 50 per cent of patients, with 15 per cent having considerable disagreement (Browning, 1997). Bacteriological culture of the discharge is usually not warranted. Likewise straight radiology is rarely helpful. Some surgeons find CT scanning helpful in identifying anatomical variants and potential fistulae of the lateral semicircular canals, though the sensitivity involved in assessing the latter is poor.

Management

Surgical

Surgery should be the mainstay of management in those with recurrent or persistently active chronic otitis media, irrespective of whether there is mucosal disease or cholesteatoma. In experienced surgical hands, ∼ 90 per cent of ears operated upon will become permanently inactive with no deterioration in the hearing. These results cannot be matched by medical therapy (*Table 10.4*). The surgical options are varied and are discussed in other texts (see, for example, Tos, 1993). Medical

Table 10.2 Percentage of patients with active chronic otitis media reporting frequency of ear discharge, discharge being visible and mopping

	Daily	Sometimes	Rarely	Severe	Tolerable	None
Frequency of discharge	47	32	21			
Runs out	41	35	24			
Dry crust on ear	50	28	21			
Wets pillow	37	25	38			
Frequency of mopping	69	24	4			
Smell				80	10	10
Concern with smell				68	12	20

(After Browning, 1997b)

therapy has a role in the treatment of occasional activity, prior to surgery and in those that decline surgery.

Medical

The only proven medical therapy is antibiotic/steroid ear drops (Browning *et al.*, 1983; Picozzi *et al.*, 1993; Browning, 1988) (*Table 10.4*). This only applies to ears with mucosal disease and requires debris to be removed by aural toilet so that the medication can reach the mucosa. A spray will achieve better distribution of the medication in an open mastoid cavity (McGarry and Swan, 1992) and many patients find it easier to use than drops. The main drawback of topical therapy is that even if it is effective, recurrent activity occurs in 40 per cent of hospital patients after a lapse of 6 weeks (Browning *et al.*, 1988). Another drawback of such medication is the potential, rather than real, risk of ototoxicity as they usually contain aminoglyco-

Table 10.4 Medical management of active mucosal chronic otitis media

Spontaneous resolution (4–6 weeks)	20%
Boric and iodine	20%
Systemic antibiotics	30%
Topical antibiotics	30%
Topical antibiotics with steroids	65%

(After Browning *et al.*, 1983 and 1988)

sides (see p. 70). Hence, as stated above, topical antibiotic steroid drops are really only indicated for those with occasional discharge, those that are not bothered by the discharge and those that are unfit for surgery. They can also be used prior to surgery to lessen the activity and make the operation technically easier to perform.

Otosclerosis

Outcomes

Disease complications

The commonest complication is a progressive conductive hearing impairment of up to an air–bone gap of 60 dB. Some suggest that cochlear involvement by the otosclerotic foci is possible, causing an additional sensorineural component (see p. 56).

Symptoms

Hearing impairment with or without tinnitus is the main symptom.

Investigation

Otosclerosis is the presumptive diagnosis when the tympanic membrane is normal and there is a conductive impairment. Tympanometry is of no value in confirming the diagnosis (see p. 40) but can be helpful in excluding otitis media with effusion (see p. 138). In the future it is likely that, with increasingly sophisticated CT scanning, otosclerotic foci will be identified with a high sensitivity and specificity. This is not the case at present.

Management

Surgery

Stapedotomy in experienced hands will eliminate the conductive impairment in the majority of ears (*Table 10.5*).

Medical

Fluoride therapy is a controversial issue particularly as the biochemical and pathological processes in otosclerosis are poorly understood. Histologically the foci are similar to

Table 10.5 Example of audit of hearing outcomes following stapedotomy for otosclerosis

Air bone gap (dB) 0.5, 1, 2 kHz	Mean	SD	≤ 0	1–10	11–20	Percentage 21–30	31–40	41–50	50+
Pre-operative	36	10	0	0	8	24	37	23	7
Post-operative (Post-op BC)	11	10	11	51	26	7	6		
Post-operative (Pre-op BC)	9	17	30	42	11	9	5	2	1

Change (negative values indicate poorer hearing)	Mean	SD	< −20	dB better −19– −10	−9–0	Percentage change 1–10	11–20	dB worse 21–30	30+
Bone conduction dB 0.5, 1, 2 kHz	−1.7	13.6	1	16	57	23	1	1	1
Air conduction dB 4 kHz	−18.0	15.6	52	31	13	43	0	1	1

(Swan, I.R.C., unpublished data, 1997)
BC = bone conduction

immature bone and fluoride in theory might stabilize the condition. There are few well-controlled studies that have looked at whether progression of the conductive or sensorineural impairment is affected by therapy. To date, the evidence is that it probably has a marginal effect (Bretlau *et al.*, 1989) but that is not necessary to give fluorides where there are high natural or treated levels of fluoride in the drinking water (Vartiainen and Vartiainen, 1996).

Otitis media with effusion

Otitis media with effusion (OME) in adults is considerably less common than in children and has been less studied. This is unfortunate because it is not uncommon in adults and its aetiology and management outcomes are likely to be different from those in children.

recognize that they would like to be able to auto-inflate their ears but cannot.

Outcomes

Disease complications

These are assumed to be the same as in childhood OME, that is healed and chronic otitis media.

Symptoms

Hearing impairment is the main symptom. This is not so fluctuant as in children. Patients often

Investigation

Otoscopy, audiometry and tympanometry have similar roles as in children (see p. 137). Some cases may be secondary to chronic rhinosinusitis which may be suspected from the symptoms of rhinorrhoea, blocked nose and facial discomfort. Rigid nasendoscopy rather than radiology is used to confirm this diagnosis. In Caucasians the incidence of nasopharyngeal tumours is so low that endoscopy of the post-nasal space with biopsy is not routinely indicated to exclude this.

Management

Non-medical

The first line of management should be auto-inflation. Many adults cannot perform a Valsalva manoeuvre and should be taught to use an Otovent balloon. Aeration of the middle ear can be achieved in many with this, which avoids surgery or a hearing aid.

Surgery

Because OME is a more protracted condition in adults than in children (Dempster and Swan, 1988), long term rather than short term ventilation tubes are warranted. Fortunately, second-ary infection with these seems less common than in children. A proportion of adults with OME will have a mixed hearing impairment and will merit the provision of a hearing aid even if the conductive impairment is managed with ventilation tubes. In such cases there is an argument for only giving an aid, particularly if they are elderly.

Medical

Patients with associated chronic rhinosinusitis should be treated appropriately which may or may not affect the OME. As in children the role of antibiotics, nasal decongestants, systemic decongestants and mucolytics is unproven.

Acute otitis media

Acute otitis media (AOM) is primarily a condition of young children (0–4 years). As such its discussion is slightly out of place in this chapter which primarily deals with adult external and middle ear conditions. Acute otitis media can occur in adults but is uncommon. There is considerable literature on the condition in children and there is currently no reason to think that the findings will not also apply to adults.

Outcomes

Disease complications

These can be classified as: (1) complications due to spread of the infection during the acute stage; (2) medium term; (3) long term.

(1) In developed countries, complications due to spread of the infection are thankfully relatively uncommon, this being as much due to improvements in general health and a better home environment as to antibiotic therapy. Acute mastoiditis occurs in about 0.04 per cent of episodes (van Buchem et al., 1981). Meningitis and Bezhold's abscesses in the neck are even rarer.

(2) The main medium term complication is otitis media with effusion (OME) which persists for 3 months or longer in about 33 per cent of ears. No randomized controlled trial as yet shows that antibiotic therapy during the acute episode affects the occurrence of OME.

(3) The long term complication is chronic otitis media. This is a postulated rather than a proven one, it being difficult to see what could cause chronic otitis media apart from acute otitis media and otitis media with effusion. Unfortunately it is not possible to predict which of the many children that have acute otitis media are likely to progress to chronic otitis media and certainly there is no evidence that therapy including surgery affects this.

Symptoms

The classic picture is of a young infant, 1–2 years old, with an upper respiratory tract infection waking up in the night crying, feverish and rubbing its ear. Apart from acute otitis media, the differential diagnosis includes negative middle ear pressure and urinary tract or chest infections.

Investigation

Otoscopy is the key to diagnosis, but this can be difficult due to the fractiousness of the child and sometimes wax in the canal. Interpretation of the findings is also not easy. Most fevered, crying children, for whatever reason, have a reddish, inflamed tympanic membrane. This will usually be bilateral. Acute otitis media is more commonly unilateral and early in the condition the pars tensa may be retracted due to negative middle ear pressure. This later becomes bulging because of middle ear pus under pressure which in some cases will rupture the pars tensa. In theory tympanometry could be an aid to diagnosis but is infrequently available. Pneumatic otoscopy may be helpful.

Management

Medical

As with any painful condition analgesics should be prescribed (e.g. Calpol). Because of the fever, adequate fluid intake is encouraged and body cooling by conventional means is carried out. The majority (60 per cent) of children will be better within 24 hours (Del Mar et al., 1997). For the 14 per cent that still have otalgia 2–7 days later, antibiotics have an effect on the pain. Hence the strategy proposed, mainly by van Buchem et al. (1981 and 1985), that antibiotics be reserved for children that are not better after 24–48 hours, seems an appropriate one. Amoxycillin is currently the antibiotic of choice. Unfortunately, as mentioned earlier, antibiotics given in the acute stage have no proven effect on recurrence of AOM or the persistence of OME.

Bone-conduction aids including bone-anchored hearing aids

Candidature

A definite indication for a bone-conduction aid is a patient without a pinna or external auditory canal to hold the mould of a conventional hearing aid. Fortunately bilateral congenital atresias are uncommon. Acquired atresias due to chronic stenosing otitis externa are also relatively uncommon and surgery to create a canal is often unsuccessful in the long term. A much larger group are patients in whom a bone-conduction aid is one possible option rather than the only option, as applies to patients with active chronic otitis who are non-responsive to medical or surgical management. They can wear a conventional aid but some consider the mould of this to exacerbate activity and increase the visibility and smell of the discharge.

Types of aid

Conventional bone-conduction aids have a headband to hold the vibrator in place on the mastoid which is both uncomfortable and cosmetically unappealing to wear. The sound processor can be worn on a belt or a behind-the-ear aid can be adapted and fitted to the headband. Unfortunately the sound heard with these systems is often distorted.

A bone-anchored hearing aid (BAHA) overcomes all these problems (Hakansson et al., 1990). It requires a small operation to tap a titanium screw into the mastoid bone with an area of non-hair-bearing skin around it. Three months later, once this is osteo-integrated, an ear-level BAHA can be attached percutaneously to an abutment attached to the screw. A BAHA is essentially a hearing aid that vibrates rather than providing amplified sound. Because the skull is directly vibrated, the amount of energy is greater and the distortion less than with conventional bone-conduction aids. Unfortunately, though superior to conventional bone-conduction aids, the amount of gain available is less than with air-conduction aids. Hence it is essential that the bone-conduction thresholds are better than the maximum frequency-specific thresholds specified (*Table 10.6*) for a patient to benefit. The body aid in this table is a more powerful sound processor and is attached by an electric cord to a vibrator attached to the peg.

Several studies have shown that the aided thresholds and speech reception are invariably superior in comparison to those using conventional bone-conduction aids (Browning and Gatehouse, 1994; Mylanus *et al.*, 1994).

Table 10.6 Maximum not-masked bone-conduction thresholds for candidacy for a bone-anchored hearing aid (BAHA)

	0.25 kHz	0.5 kHz	1 kHz	2 kHz	3 kHz	4 kHz
Ear level	25	35	50	55	60	60
Body	25	45	60	65	70	70

(After Gatehouse and Browning, 1990)

This is not the case when a comparison is made with air-conduction aids. Here the aided thresholds and speech reception may or may not be superior with the BAHA. There is no doubt that a BAHA is very comfortable to wear but it does have the disadvantage that the peg needs to be kept clean and sometimes granulations can develop around it. Fortunately, loss of the titanium screw because of non-integration is uncommon. The final and not least aspect to consider, is the cost. Apart from the surgical costs, the aid and the titanium implants are more expensive (around £2000 in 1997) than air-conduction aids by a large margin. Along with the fact that a BAHA is not always acoustically superior to an air-conduction aid, this means that the decision to provide a BAHA can be a difficult one in patients in whom a bone-conduction aid is not the only option.

Disability associated with a hearing impairment

The disability an individual patient may have as a result of a hearing impairment can be predicted from the audiogram, measured by various audiometric methods or ascertained by questioning the patient. These three methods can be used to assess the reduction in disability (i.e. benefit from management) with a hearing aid or surgery. At present most decisions are made by prediction from the audiogram along with some limited, fairly unstructured questioning of the patient. The current non-use of audiometric methods is primarily due to their unavailability except in research centres and their lack of proven applicability to clinical settings. Audiometric methods combine listening with vision and assess speech understanding in backgrounds of noise as well as the ability to localize sounds. The main disadvantage of predicting the disability from the audiogram is a lack of knowledge of a particular patient's listening requirements. Thus, although it is known that the overall disability is largely determined by the hearing in the better ear, this is less the case in a background of noise. How often a

listener is in various listening situations and how important it is for them to hear in such situations will influence the degree of disability. *Table 10.7* lists the commoner listening situations most people encounter, and the time spent in them. This table applies to patients being fitted with a hearing aid and will be different in those undergoing middle ear surgery. What it shows is that it is important to concentrate on what matters to a specific patient, there being many other situations that only apply to a subgroup, such as listening at

Table 10.7 Report of situations that cause awareness of a hearing disability and time spent in these situations in patients being fitted with a hearing aid

Disability situation	%	Time spent
Conversation in quiet	83	
Conversation in noise	95	
Television	83	21 hours per week
Meetings/clubs	70	4 hours per week
Telephone use	55	5 minutes per day

(GRI clinic data)

church. Various questionnaires have been designed to evaluate hearing disability and have to date mainly been used to identify residual disability after hearing aid fitting.

In the surgical domain, fuller discussion of the objectives and likely outcomes with patients and their relatives are increasingly being called for. Purchasers are paying increasing attention to the benefits and costs of intervention. Hence surgeons increasingly have to know the technical results of their surgery, the likely outcomes and the potential benefit in terms of relief of disability.

Outcomes of surgery for hearing

When middle ear surgery is performed to improve the patient's hearing it can be technically successful to varying degrees. Unfortunately, sometimes there may be secondary inner ear damage. The literature contains many papers where the world experts report their results. Assuming that these reports are honest, the average surgeon is unlikely to achieve the same results. Not everybody can be a world expert so it is essential that each surgeon audits their own results. This can help in the discussion with the patient, where the real chances of the various outcomes rather than hypothetical ones can be quoted. There is a tendency for some surgeons to say that they know their results without auditing them. Of course this is nonsense, as anyone who has audited their results knows. For example, everyone will say that it is routine to carry out an audiogram post-operatively. When it comes to looking for them in the case-sheet it is another matter. Finally, it is important to be able to predict the likely benefit from surgery. This is not necessarily the same as the technical benefit as will be discussed later.

Technical results

In surgery to improve hearing the technical objective is to reduce the conductive defect as much as possible without making the hearing worse by causing a sensorineural impairment. An audiometric measure of each of these parameters is required from the pure tone audiogram. What data to monitor are debated and are likely to be different in research settings where finer measures are perhaps required

and more threshold data may be available. In the UK, air-conduction thresholds at 0.5, 1, 2 and 4 kHz are usually available, but 3 and 8 kHz less frequently so. Bone conduction thresholds at 0.5, 1, 2 and often 4 kHz are usually available but seldom at 3 kHz. American (Committee of AAOO, 1965 and 1995) and Japanese (Sakai, 1994) recommendations have been published but are not ideal, having been arrived at by committees. In the earlier American and the current Japanese recommendations, measures of technical success and patient benefit are intermixed. The later American recommendations (*Table 10.8*) are much clearer, doing away with the controversy discussed below as to which bone-conduction thresholds to use and recommending that the air–bone gap be calculated from the thresholds recorded on a specific occasion. Unfortunately they recommend that thresholds at 3 kHz be used in the averages along with 0.5, 1 and 2 kHz but these are not routinely available in most patients. This they acknowledge but recommend it for the future. However, averaging the thresholds over 0.5, 1, 2 and

Table 10.8 Guidelines for results of treatment for conductive hearing loss

(1) Air–bone gap at 0.6, 1, 2 and 3 kHz at 1 year
(2) Number of dB closure of air–bone gap at 1 year
(3) Change in bone-conduction at 3 and 4 kHz

Report mean, SD and range
Air–bone gaps in 10 dB bins

(From American Academy of Otolaryngology and Head and Neck Surgery, 1994)

4 kHz is unlikely to be materially different (Berliner *et al.*, 1996).

A standard method is important to allow comparisons for audit purposes. Making comparisons between different techniques will always be difficult, for example stapedectomy versus stapedotomy, because any differences are likely to be small and numbers have to be large to show statistical significance.

Measures of change in the conduction defect

The magnitude of the conduction defect is best measured by the air–bone gap, which by convention is a three frequency average over 0.5, 1 and 2 kHz. Some advocate a four frequency average over 0.5, 1, 2 and either 3 or 4 kHz. Both air- and bone-conduction thresholds should be available pre- and post-operatively. The main debate is whether to use the pre-operative, the post-operative or the better of the two bone-conduction averages. If the pre-operative thresholds are used, the residual conductive defect is likely to be underestimated. The post-operative average can be better than the pre-operative one because of the Carhart effect or it can be poorer because of sensorineural damage. If the post-operative

thresholds are used, sensorineural losses associated with lessening of the conduction defect will be missed. Using the better of the two lessens both deficiencies.

This is exemplified by taking the pre-operative audiogram in *Figure 10.1* with the two possible outcomes in *Figures 10.2* and *10.3*. In both, the air–bone gap has been closed but the results are very different (*Table 10.9*).

Whilst the above makes for an interesting debate, the question is 'Does it really matter'? Two papers have looked at what the differences are in patients following stapes surgery (Berliner *et al.*, 1996) and following tympanoplasty (Goldenberg and Berliner, 1995). No matter how the results were analysed there was no real difference in the outcomes in tympanoplasty surgery. This was not the case with stapes surgery, mainly because the Carhart effect was more likely to be evident and damage at 4 kHz more likely. Because of the wealth of data involved, these two papers from several centres are perhaps the best sources to use for comparison for audit purposes. Unfortunately, they only report mean data with standard deviations and do not have data as recommended for 10 dB bins (see *Table 10.5*, p. 102).

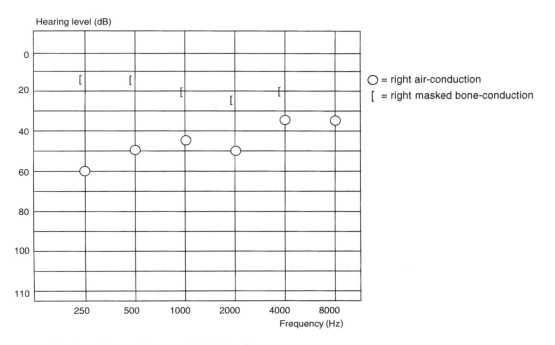

Figure 10.1 Ear with a moderate conductive impairment

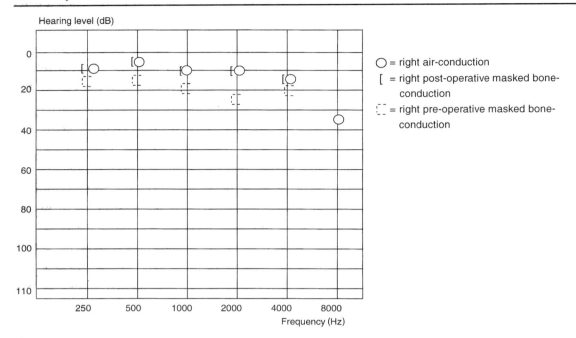

Figure 10.2 A good post-operative result from surgery on an ear with the pre-operative audiogram in *Figure 10.1*. The air–bone gap has been overclosed using the pre-operative bone-conduction thresholds. These are better post-operatively because of the Carhart effect

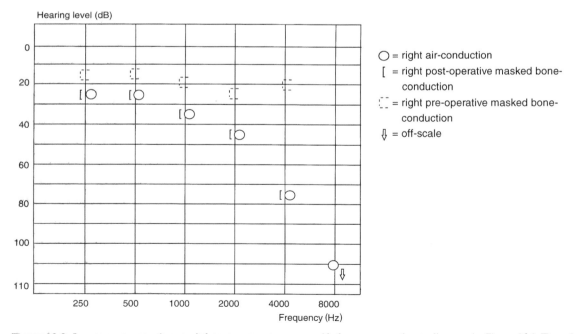

Figure 10.3 A poor post-operative result from surgery on an ear with the pre-operative audiogram in *Figure 10.1*. Though the air–bone gap has been closed using the post-operative bone-conduction thresholds, these are poorer than pre-operative because of inner ear damage as evidenced by a sensorineural impairment. The air–bone gap in comparison to the pre-operative bone-conduction is of course not closed but it is smaller (28 dB reduced to 15 dB). The patient will obviously not benefit from this

Table 10.9 Thresholds from *Figures 10.1, 10.2* and *10.3*

		0.5 kHz	*1 kHz*	*2 kHz*	*Total*	*Average*
Figure 10.1, pre-operative	AC	50	45	50	95	32
	BC	15	20	25	60	20
Figure 10.2, post-operative	AC	5	10	10	25	8
	BC	5	10	10	25	8
Figure 10.3, post-operative	AC	25	35	45	105	35
	BC	25	35	45	105	35

	Figure 10.2	*Figure 10.3*
Pre-operative ABG	12	12
Post-operative ABG		
Using:		
Pre-operative BC	-16	$+3$
Post-operative BC	0	0
Better BC	-16	0

AC = air conduction; BC = bone conduction; ABG = air-bone gap

Measures of damage to the hearing

Surgical damage to the inner ear is more likely at the higher frequencies and hence worsening of the air-conduction threshold at 8 kHz would be the most sensitive measure. Damage localized to this frequency is not as detrimental to the hearing of speech as damage at 4 kHz. Hence worsening of the hearing at 4 kHz by air conduction is a better clinical measure, though it will include patients whose hearing is worse due to an increase in the conductive defect as well as those suffering sensorineural damage. To distinguish between such cases is not clinically important, what matters is the overall number. In the example shown (*Figures 10.1 and 10.3*) the 4 kHz air-conduction thresholds are poorer by 40 dB post-operatively.

As well as reporting for 4 kHz, the lower frequencies should also be reported. As explained previously (see p. 43) the bone-conduction thresholds are affected by a conductive defect. They may get better with surgical correction of the conductive defect. If they get poorer it is almost certainly because of inner ear damage. As the pre- and post-operative thresholds over 0.5, 1 and 2 kHz have already been used to measure the air–bone gap it seems reasonable to report any change for the worse in these as a measure of sensorineural damage. Thus in the previous example (*Figures 10.1 and 10.3*) there is a worsening of the bone-conduction average by 15 dB.

Table 10.5 (see p. 102) is an example of how the technical results of middle ear surgery should be reported, in this case taking stapedotomy as an example. In this case it will be noted that the mean results are less meaningful than the distribution of the results in 10 dB bins.

Patient benefit

The main reason why patient benefit is not equatable to technical results is that a patient has two ears and surgery at any one time is on one ear. Frequently this involves the poorer hearing ear, for the very valid reason that, in the event of the hearing becoming poorer, the patient will be consequently less disabled. Unfortunately the contrary is also the case, that if the hearing is improved the benefit will be less than if the same improvement had occurred in the better hearing ear.

Formerly the American guidelines recommended that the air-conduction levels be reported post-operatively as a measure of hearing. This is valid if one wants to assess the likely post-operative monaural disability. It is not a measure of change, for which one needs to make a comparison between the pre-operative and the post-operative air-conduction thresholds.

Whilst results for the ear operated upon have some meaning, the main determinant of overall hearing disability is the hearing in the better hearing ear. This is because in most circumstances, even when sound originates on the side of the poorer ear, it will be heard by the better ear attenuated by 15 dB in quiet and 45 dB in noise. Thus, taking Patient A in *Figure 10.4* with unilateral otosclerosis, the hearing in the left ear is normal and there is a moderate

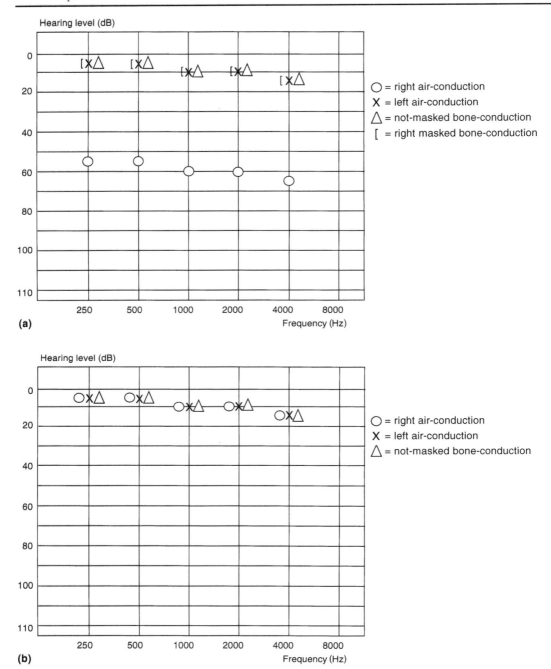

Figure 10.4 (a) Patient A, pre-operative: Glasgow plot area 2. (b) Patient A, post-operative: Glasgow plot area 1. (see Figures 10.10 and 10.11)

conductive impairment in the right ear. This patient will only be really disabled in a background of noise when a speaker is on the poorer hearing side. This is in contrast to Pa-

tient B with bilateral moderate hearing loss due to otosclerosis in *Figure 10.5a*. This patient will be disabled in most listening circumstances. The magnitude of the air–bone gap in

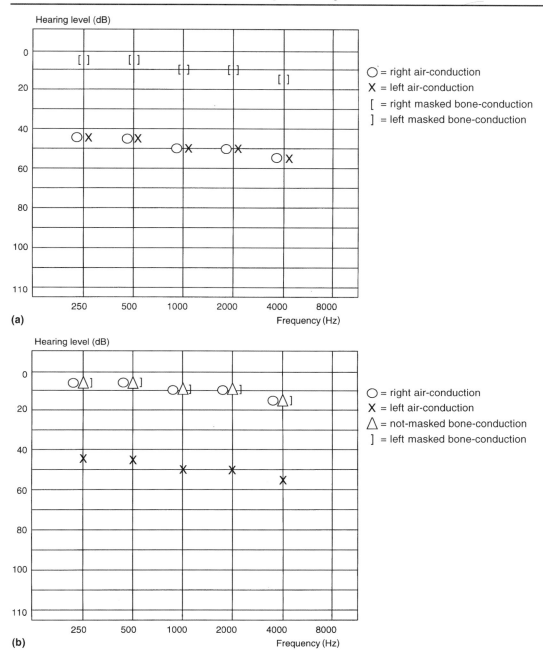

Figure 10.5 (a) Patient B, pre-operative: Glasgow plot area 5. (b) Patient B, post-operative: Glasgow plot area 3 (see Figures 10.10 and 10.11)

each patient is the same and if closed by surgery the technical results in each patient will be the same (*Figure 10.4b* and *Figure 10.5b*) but the benefit will be different. Patient A (*Figure 10.4b*) will not now have difficulty in hearing in a background of noise when the speaker is on their bad side. Patient B (*Figure 10.5b*) will now be able to hear normally in most circumstances, the exception being in a noisy background with speech on their poorer side. Common sense would suggest that Patient B would report more benefit than Patient

A and this has been confirmed scientifically (Browning, 1997). After a period of time Patient B might want their other ear operated on and, if this was technically successful in closing the air–bone gap, they would then have bilaterally normal hearing after the second operation. Experience of such patients having a second side stapedectomy is that they are less delighted with the second operation than the first.

Up until now we have solely discussed patients with a pure conductive hearing impairment in whom it is possible to make the hearing in one ear normal. How is this changed in patients with mixed hearing impairments? Patient C has a severe mixed impairment in the right ear and a mild sensorineural impairment in the left (*Figure 10.6a*). Patient D has a bilateral severe mixed impairment (*Figure 10.7a*). Assuming that neither patient wears a hearing aid before or after surgery, and the air–bone gap is closed in each patient (*Figures 10.6 and 10.7b*), it is extremely likely that Patient D will report more benefit than Patient C.

So the conclusion is that patients with a pre-operative symmetric impairment are likely to report greater benefit than those with an asymmetric impairment. This is primarily because the operation has improved the hearing level in their better hearing ear rather than in their poorer hearing ear.

The next question to be addressed is which, of Patients B and D, is likely to report the greater benefit? Convention has it that Patient B is the more likely because their operated on better hearing ear is now 'normal' in comparison to Patient D whose operated on, better hearing ear is still impaired (Smyth, 1985; Toner and Smyth, 1993). The contrary view is that it is not the achieving of a specific threshold that matters (e.g. 30 dB HL to constitute normality) but how much the hearing is improved in the operated on ear (Browning, 1997b). Thus, in this instance Patient D would report just as much benefit as Patient B, because the air-conduction thresholds have been improved by an equal amount in each patient.

Now, what about the comparison between Patient A and Patient C? Patient A starts with a mild disability and has none post-operatively. Patient C starts with a greater disability but still has a mild disability post-operatively. The reported benefit is likely to be similar, provided Patient C is counselled before the operation

not to expect to have normal hearing but only to have symmetrical hearing.

So far only patients with a bilateral symmetrical impairment have been considered where the magnitude of the air–bone gap in each ear is the same. A bilateral conductive impairment where the air–bone gaps are different is more frequent and gives rise to a bilateral but asymmetrical impairment. The bone-conduction thresholds may (Patient E, *Figure 10.8a*) or may not be normal (Patient F, *Figure 10.9a*). In both instances closing the air–bone gap makes the operated on ear the better hearing ear. In one instance the operated on ear beats a certain level of normality (30 dB HL) and the other does not. What appears to measure benefit in these circumstances is the magnitude of the change rather than the reaching of a certain level.

Glasgow plot

It is with this concept of grouping patients into different pre- and post-operative categories that the Glasgow plot was devised (*Figure 10.10*). The mean air-conduction thresholds in the non-operated on ear are plotted on the horizontal axis and the ear to be operated on, on the vertical axis. Thirty dB HL is taken as the level of 'normal' hearing thresholds. Patients who fall into the rectangular areas 2 and 3 will have one normal hearing ear. Patients falling into the square consisting of areas 4–6 will have bilateral, impaired thresholds. Within this square the two diagonal lines delineate area 5 which includes patients with a bilateral hearing impairment whose thresholds are symmetrical, i.e. within 10 dB of each other. The triangular areas 4 and 6 indicate patients with a bilateral hearing impairment whose thresholds are asymmetrical, i.e. greater than 10 dB apart. It is accepted that surgery should not usually be performed on a better hearing ear, and most patients pre-operatively will fall into areas 2, 5 or 6.

Those in area 2 have a unilateral impairment such as in *Figure 10.4a*. Patients in area 5 have a bilateral symmetrical hearing impairment such as in *Figures 10.5a* and *10.7a*. Patients in area 6 have a bilateral but asymmetrical impairment such as in *Figures 10.6a*, *10.8a* and *10.9a*. Post-operatively, if surgery improves the air-conduction thresholds, the patient could

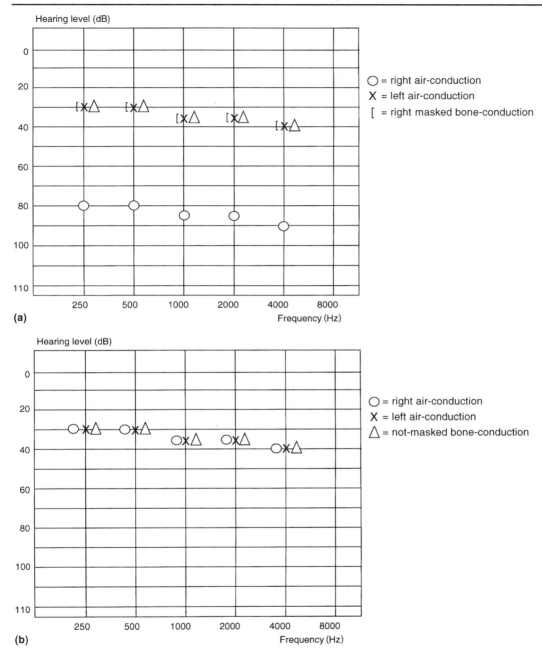

Figure 10.6 (a) Patient C, pre-operative: Glasgow plot area 6. (b) Patient C, post-operative: Glasgow plot area 5 (see Figures 10.10 and 10.11)

change category, i.e. a patient with a unilateral conductive impairment in area 2 could, post-operatively, have bilateral normal thresholds in area 1 (*Figure 10.4b*). A patient with pre-operative bilateral symmetrical but impaired thresholds in area 5 could, post-operatively, have a unilateral normal ear in area 3 (*Figure 10.5b*) or the operated on ear could become the better ear, but still be impaired in area 4 (*Figure 10.7b*). Patients with a bilateral but asymmetrical impairment in area 6 could, post-operatively, have unilateral normal thresh-

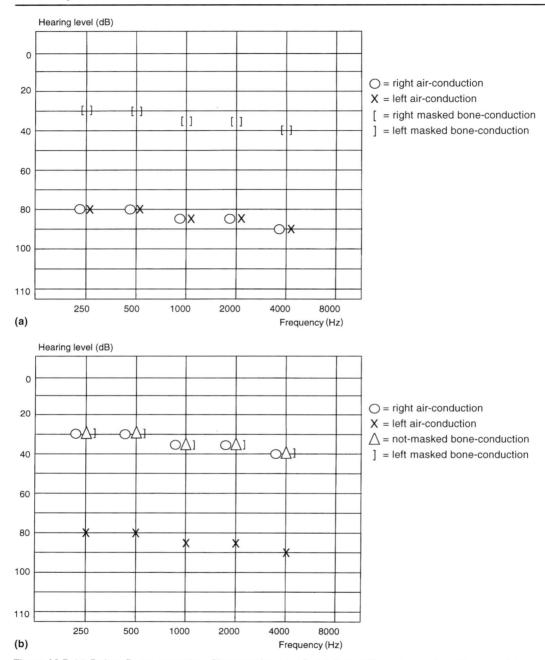

Figure 10.7 (a) Patient D, pre-operative: Glasgow plot area 5. (b) Patient D, post-operative: Glasgow plot area 4 (see Figures 10.10 and 10.11)

olds in area 3 (*Figure 10.8b*) or the operated on ear could become the better hearing ear but still be impaired in area 4 (*Figure 10.9b*) or symmetrical but impaired thresholds in area 5 could be achieved (*Figure 10.6b*). All these six different pre-/post-operative audiometric changes that can occur with technically successful surgery are plotted in *Figure 10.11*.

When experienced surgeons are questioned about the likely reported benefit from

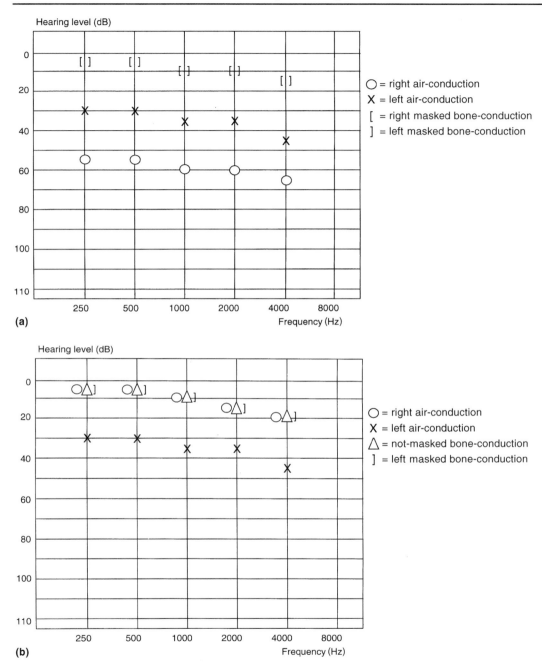

Figure 10.8 (a) Patient E, pre-operative: Glasgow plot area 6. (b) Patient E, post-operative: Glasgow plot area 3 (see Figures 10.10 and 10.11)

these various categories, there is a variety of opinion but they all consider that the benefits are likely to be different even though the surgery has been technically successful. In general they rank the gaining of normal hearing

thresholds above the gaining of symmetrical hearing (Browning, 1997b).

When patients are asked about the benefit to their general health as opposed to the effect on their hearing, again there is a large difference

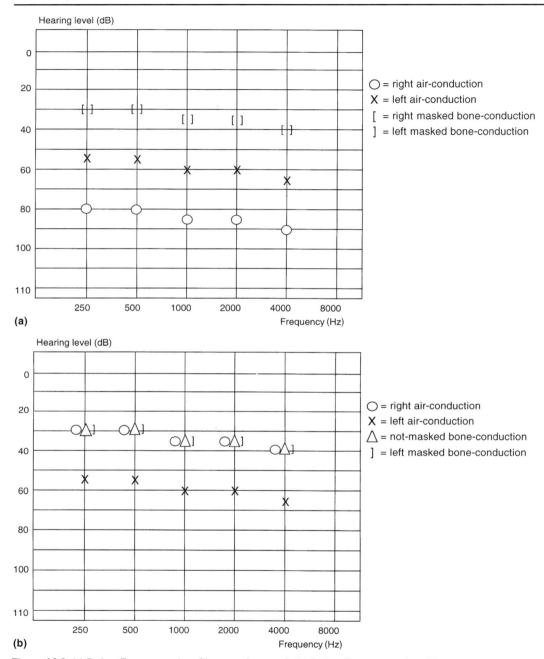

Figure 10.9 (a) Patient F, pre-operative: Glasgow plot area 6. (b) Patient F, post-operative: Glasgow plot area 4 (see Figures 10.10 and 10.11)

depending on which pre-operative hearing category they fall into. Patients with a bilateral asymmetric pre-operative impairment report greater benefit than those with a bilateral symmetric impairment, who in turn report greater benefit than those with a unilateral impairment.

This order of rank is with the proviso that in those with a bilateral hearing impairment the operation makes the operated on ear the better hearing ear. Thus operating on a patient with a unilateral mixed impairment when the other ear has a sensorineural impairment (*Figure*

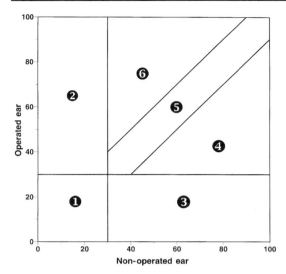

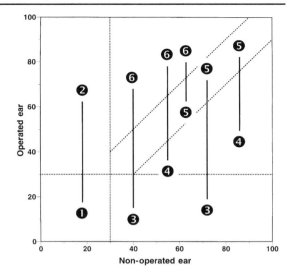

Figure 10.10 Glasgow plot (see Figures 10.4–10.9 for details of numbered areas)

Figure 10.11 Pre-/post-operative audiometric changes in Glasgow plot

10.6a) is unlikely to be considered particularly beneficial. Within each group it is the magnitude of the change in the hearing that measures benefit rather than the achieving of a certain

hearing level such as 30 dB HL. When one thinks about this it is understandable. It is the size of the reduction in disability rather than the residual disability that matters.

■ Conclusions

• The methods of management of specific external and middle ear conditions are too many to summarize here. The following conclusions are applicable to most patients with a conductive hearing impairment irrespective of the aetiology.

• Bone conduction aids are an option to consider along with conventional aids in individuals with a conductive component to their impairment.

• Bone-anchored hearing aids are acoustically superior to conventional bone-conduction aids, more comfortable to wear and cosmetically more appealing. Certain minimum bone-conduction thresholds must be present for aiding to be beneficial.

• Bone-conduction aids are mandatory in those with bilateral congenital or acquired atresias of the external auditory canal.

• They are optional in those with a discharging ear resulting from otitis externa or active chronic otitis media. In such patients the benefit gained with the aid may or may not be better than with conventional aids.

• In ear surgery audit of a surgeon's technical results is important because of the considerable variation there is in such results. This allows the real chance of technical success to be discussed with the patient rather than a hypothetical one.

• The technical results regarding the hearing should report the means and standard deviation, along with details of:

(1) the pre- and post-operative air–bone gap over 0.5, 1 and 2 kHz using the pre-operative bone conduction;

(2) the pre- and post-operative bone conduction over 0.5, 1 and 2 kHz;
(3) the pre- and post-operative air conduction at 4 kHz.

These should be reported as mean dB with standard deviations. The results should also be reported in 10 dB bins.

• Patient benefit from surgery to improve the hearing depends primarily on the magnitude of the change in air-conduction thresholds and the pre-operative category of the hearing.
• The Glasgow plot categorizes patients into one of three pre-operative categories: unilateral impairment, bilateral symmetric impairment and bilateral asymmetric impairment. This is in the order of increasing benefit from improvement in the air-conduction thresholds.

• The gaining of a certain level of hearing (e.g. 30 dB) which equates with normal does not appear to be a determinant of perceived benefit.
• Benefit is determined by the magnitude of the change in air-conduction thresholds and depends on the pre-operative classification of their binaural hearing.

Further reading

Browning, G.G. (1997) Do patients and surgeons agree? Gordon Smyth Memorial Lecture. *Clinical Otolaryngology*, **22**, 485–496.
Tos, M. (1993) *Manual of Middle Ear Surgery*, Volume 1. Approaches: Myringoplasty, Ossiculoplasty and Tympanoplasty. Thieme Verlag, Stuttgart.

11 Management of adult severe, profound and total hearing impairments

A severe impairment is defined as a pure tone average over 0.5, 1, 2 and 4 kHz between 70 and 89 dB HL, a profound impairment as one between 90 and 109 dB HL, and a total impairment as one worse than 110 dB HL. Though such impairments affect only 1 per cent of the adult population they constitute 12 per cent of the hearing-impaired population seeking advice (GRI clinic data), and their management is particularly time-consuming and difficult. This is so for several interrelated reasons.

Patient characteristics

Type of impairment

Two-thirds (65 per cent) of patients with a severe or profound hearing impairment have a mixed impairment (McClymont and Browning, 1991). This is usually because a patient has a conductive impairment due to chronic otitis media or otosclerosis to which is added an age-related sensorineural impairment. Less frequently the middle ear disease or the management thereof is the cause of the sensorineural component. Many of these patients will also have ears which are intermittently active due to chronic otitis media, frequently with an open mastoid cavity. The other third of the patients have a sensorineural impairment. None has a pure conductive impairment as it is rare to have an air–bone gap greater than 60 dB.

Age

Because the majority have an age-related sensorineural component to their impairment, the average age of this population is 68 years (Giles *et al.*, 1996). Hence, their lifestyle, degree of motivation and physical limitations are different from those of a younger population with a pure conductive impairment.

Disability

Conversational speech is usually around 65 dB A. Hence, its comprehension by those with a severe or profound impairment in their better ear relies mainly on speech-reading. Thus, unless aided, speech is incomprehensible when the speaker's face is not visible.

Environmental noises such as traffic and alerting bells may also not be heard. Another related problem is hearing their own voice and this is especially so in those with poor sensori-neural thresholds. Without this auditory feedback a patient's speech becomes flat and of an inappropriate volume.

Audiometric assessment

As in all patients with a hearing impairment, the basis of assessment is pure tone audiometry (Chapter 3) but in this group of patients it can be difficult. It is usually possible to be fairly certain what the air-conduction thresholds are in the better hearing ear, but frequently this is all that can be ascertained with any degree of certainty. This is primarily because of the limited bone-conduction output of audiometers and difficulties in masking due to the limit of output of masking sound of around 115 dB. *Figures 11.1–11.5* are some examples which should be read to understand some of the problems involved.

These problems do not usually significantly affect management with conventional hearing aids. The problems also do not apply to bone-conduction aids as such aids are of no potential value if not-masked bone-conduction thresholds are unrecordable. Where it does matter is if surgery to improve the hearing might be an option. Here it is: (a) important to recognize when one is operating on a sole hearing ear; (b) inadvisable to operate on a

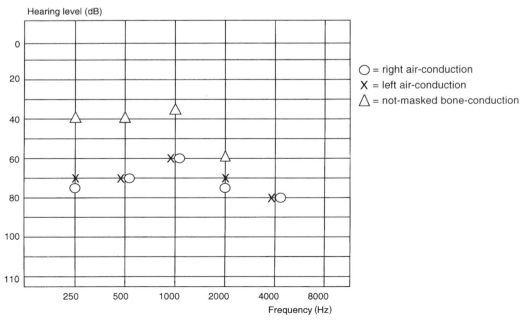

Figure 11.1 Apparent bilateral symmetric severe hearing impairment. Not-masked bone-conduction thresholds are ascertainable and must refer to at least one ear. Masking is insufficient in power to mask the air-conduction to ascertain the masked bone-conduction thresholds. Hence one ear certainly has a mixed impairment and the other ear could also have a mixed impairment or a sensorineural impairment

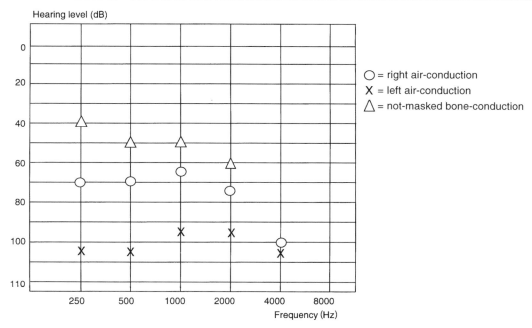

Figure 11.2 Apparent bilateral asymmetric hearing impairment. The right ear has a severe and the left a profound impairment. Masked bone conduction thresholds are not possible for the reasons given in *Figure 11.1*. On this occasion it is likely that the not-masked bone-conduction thresholds apply to the right ear because this is the better ear. The left ear could have a profound sensorineural impairment or be a 'dead' ear, as the left air-conduction thresholds could be attributable to the right bone conduction

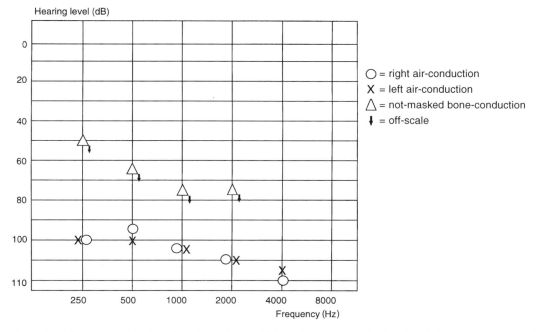

Figure 11.3 Apparent bilateral profound impairment. Not-masked bone-conduction thresholds are poorer than the maximum output of the bone-conduction vibrator. Hence, the impairment could be mixed or sensorineural in one or both ears

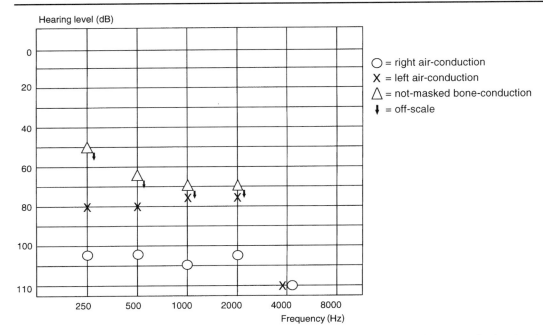

Figure 11.4 Apparent bilateral left severe and right profound impairment. Not-masked bone-conduction thresholds are poorer than the maximum output of the bone-conduction vibrator. There is likely to be left a severe sensorineural impairment. The right ear could have a mixed profound or sensorineural profound impairment or could be a 'dead' ear because of the reasons given in *Figure 11.2*

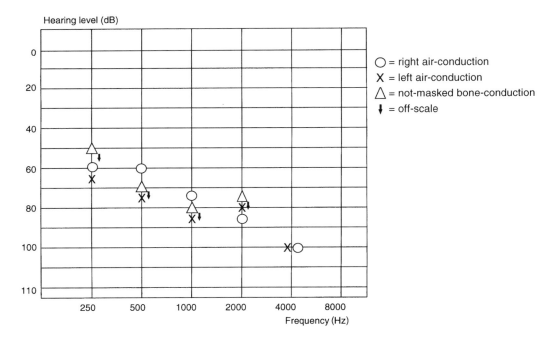

Figure 11.5 Bilateral symmetric severe sensorineural impairment. Masking is unnecessary in this case which is the only example in *Figures 11.1–11.5* where there is certainty about both the degree and type of impairment in each ear

dead ear; and (c) inadvisable to operate on an ear that does not have a conductive component. Electrocochleography is the only technique that can be used to ascertain the hearing in such ears as the electrode records from the inner ear directly and masking is unnecessary.

Management

Multiple options are available for the management of the severely impaired and the choice is often best made by a multidisciplinary team including an otologist, audiologist and a hearing therapist. A speech therapist can also be helpful, if speech production is compromised.

Air-conduction aids

Wherever possible, the patient should be encouraged to use binaural aids, mainly because of the central summation of loudness that can be achieved. Binaural aiding is accepted in the long term by about 80 per cent of this population (Day et al., 1988). Because of gain requirements, in-the-ear aids are usually inappropriate because of feedback. A wide range of behind-the-ear aids is available and nowadays it is rare to require a body aid for its greater power.

Moulds

The first task is to ensure that well-fitting moulds are available that do not allow feedback at the maximum gain that the patient will accept. This is best achieved by having a longer canal piece than normal made of soft rather than hard acrylic. Before taking an impression, the canal should be well cleared of debris and opened by pinna traction. The latter is important as many of these patients are elderly and have collapsed cartilaginous canals. Some patients will have an open mastoid cavity with a large meatoplasty which creates its own difficulties in making a mould.

Multiple attempts to get a good mould are frequently necessary and because of hardening of the mould along with expansion of the canal with time, patients should be seen at least yearly because moulds deteriorate and need to be replaced. This deterioration causes feedback and the patient avoids this by using the aid at a lesser gain than formerly.

Insertion gain

Real ear insertion gains (see p. 90) are important as they will significantly influence the choice of aids and what modifications are made to them. In some ears, islands of hearing at the lower frequencies are all that remain. Fortunately, loudness discomfort due to recruitment is not as major a problem as might be expected, mainly because feedback often occurs before this level is reached and the maximum output of the aid is insufficient to reach it.

Bone-conduction aids

Because two-thirds of the severely impaired population have a mixed hearing impairment, bone-conduction aids and in particular bone-anchored hearing aids (see p. 104) are an option to consider seriously in this group. This is particularly so because many of the ears with chronic otitis media continue to be active despite medical therapy and the fitting of moulds can be difficult because of a mastoid cavity and the associated meatoplasty. Otitis externa is another major problem which makes the wearing of an aid with an ear mould difficult, particularly because of feedback. Care has to be exercised as to whether the bone-conduction thresholds satisfy the candidature criteria to ensure benefit and even then the benefit may be less with a BAHA than with a conventional behind-the-ear aid (Snik et al., 1992).

Surgery

Although two-thirds of the patients have a mixed impairment, surgery is less frequently appropriate than might be thought. Firstly, many patients (~ 25 per cent; Giles, 1997) have already undergone surgery which has been unsuccessful in closing the air–bone gap. Secondly, in many ears, particularly those with an open mastoid cavity, no ossicular chain remains which makes successful reconstruction difficult. Thirdly, the ear that otoscopically appears the most appropriate ear for reconstructive surgery is often the better hearing ear. The inability to obtain masked bone-conduction thresholds is also a disadvantage when considering a poorer hearing ear for surgery. It might be a dead ear, particularly if it has been operated on before. It could be argued that if this is the case there is little to lose by operating on the chance that it is not a dead ear. Electrocochleography to determine the hearing status of the cochlea is the only potential way out of this dilemma.

Accessory listening devices

The severely and profoundly impaired benefit greatly from alerting devices (see p. 94). Every patient should be questioned about what type of door and telephone bells they have and where they are situated. To ask a patient whether they hear the bell is often misleading because they do not know of the occasions when they did not hear it. Alerting lights may also be helpful as an alternative. Unfortunately, the telecoil on their hearing aid often gives insufficient amplification for this group of patients.

Tinnitus

Tinnitus in this group is difficult to mask, especially if the poorer ear is affected and the patient cannot wear an aid on that side. Environmental sounds are not heard and tinnitus maskers are insufficiently powerful to be effective. Thus, one has to rely on counselling (see p. 151). In a few patients cochlear implantation can be considered. A single channel implant could be sufficient to relieve the tinnitus if there is an aidable hearing ear on the contralateral side. Unfortunately only about 50 per cent of patients get relief with an implant.

Speech-reading

It would be encouraging to think that current methods of training in speech-reading are effective but, unfortunately, this has yet to be proven. Much of the evidence that has been put forward has been from studies performed without adequate controls. This is a weakness as it is known that patients will improve their results on the various tests for speech-reading without any training because of increased familiarity with the test. Most individuals will also spontaneously learn how to benefit in speech-reading from their aid. This does not mean that training in speech-reading should be abandoned, it is just that the best form of instruction has yet to be identified. In addition, the psychological aspects of instruction should not be discounted because patients with a profound impairment require continual encouragement, but it could be that time spent on speech-reading would be better spent instructing the individuals on how best to use the hearing aids they have.

Management of the profoundly and totally impaired with cochlear implants

With experience and technical improvements in sound processing the level of hearing in the better hearing ear at which cochlear implants are appropriate is gradually falling. Initially, implants quite correctly were only indicated for those with a total impairment who could not benefit from conventional air-conduction aids. The results in such cases have frequently been better than those achieved in the profoundly impaired with conventional aids. Now cochlear implants are considered in those with a pure tone average of poorer than 105 dB HL. It is anticipated that a relaxation to 95 dB HL is likely with time (Summerfield and Marshall, 1995).

Cochlear implants

Cochlear implants stimulate residual cochlear nerve fibres with acoustic sounds which have been processed into electrical energy. They are used primarily in individuals with a profound or total sensorineural hearing loss in their better hearing ear who have not benefited from conventional hearing aids. In such individuals few hair cells remain histologically but there are still residual cochlear afferent nerve fibres which can be stimulated. Understandably the longer such a profound/total impairment has been present the less numerous the nerve fibres are likely to be because of retrograde degeneration. Many different modifications of implants are available though some are only used infrequently.

Intracochlear versus extracochlear

An intracochlear implant is inserted through the round window and fed up the turns of the cochlea. To date implants can only be fed up the first one-and-a-half turns and because the inner ear is opened such implants destroy any remaining hair cells. The surgical procedure involved is usually not technically difficult, the round window niche being accessed via a cortical mastoidectomy and a posterior tympanotomy.

Extracochlear implants stimulate the nerve fibres either via the round window membrane itself when the electrode is single channel or via the bone of the cochlea on the promontory if multichannelled. Extracochlear implants are the only option when there has been total ossification of the membranous cochlea which is not infrequent following meningitis. Theoretically such implants could be superior in frequency discrimination because they can be placed to stimulate the apex, but in practice they are less frequently used.

Multichannel versus single channel

Single channel implants were the first to be used but now they have largely been superseded by multichannel implants because of their ability to preferentially stimulate different parts of the cochlea to aid frequency discrimination. However, in practical terms, though some implants have 22 channels, only the six best are generally used.

Connection of electrode to processor

The most popular method of doing this is transcutaneous where electrical energy is inducted electromagnetically through the intact skin from one electrical coil in the processor to another at the end of the electrode which is sunk into the mastoid cortical bone. The external coil is held in place by a magnet which attracts itself to a subcutaneous magnet. The electrical energy to the external coil is fed from a body-worn sound processor.

The less frequently used percutaneous devices connect the electrode directly through the skin to a body-worn processor. Such connections have the problems of crusting and infection similar to bone-anchored hearing aids (see p. 104).

Sound processing

All systems convert sound into electrical energy and use some form of automatic gain control to compress the range of stimulation because of the considerably lesser range available in implant patients. In single channel implants the energy can only be coded in a temporal manner. In multichannel implants there is a variety of options. The whole signal can be broken up into different frequency bands. Another option is to process the sound in various ways which aid speech understanding.

Commercial models

The Nucleus multichannel device, manufactured by Cochlear, has been implanted most frequently. There are 22 channels of which up to six are used. Signal transmission utilizes speech processing and is transcutaneous. The Clarion device has 16 channels and is produced by the University of California. Multiple signal processing is possible and transmission is transcutaneous.

Assessment of suitability for implantation

Various audiometric tests have been evolved for this particular group of patients to assess the benefit from both conventional hearing aids and cochlear implants. These tests can be performed with or without speech-reading clues. In the early days caution as to who to implant was understandable and only individuals with a total impairment that did not benefit from aids were implanted. With experience it has been found that those who benefit from aids are likely to benefit even more from implants.

Hence the criterion of non-benefit from aids is being gradually dropped in favour of a certain dB HL criterion. This is currently 105 dB HL.

Non-organic hearing losses will be identified by electrophysiological tests. Electrocochleography can assess whether there are residual nerve fibres which can be stimulated but, in general, success from implantation is not related to the results of electrophysiological tests.

Patients need to be motivated to learn to use an implant and in children strong home support is essential.

Finally, the surgical technique has to be practical and CT scanning will identify cochlear abnormalities, particularly ossification, which would make it less practicable.

■ Conclusions

• A severe hearing impairment is defined as a pure tone average over 0.5, 1, 2 and 4 kHz of between 70 and 90 dB HL.
• A profound hearing impairment is an average of greater than 90 dB HL but less than 110 dB HL.
• A total hearing impairment is an average of greater than 110 dB HL.
• Adult patients with a severe or profound impairment in their better ear constitute 12 per cent of patients with an impairment managed at an otology/audiology clinic but are more time-consuming than other patients because of the problems of aiding.
• Two-thirds of patients have a mixed hearing impairment, often associated with active chronic otitis media resistant to medical and/or surgical management.
• Audiometric assessment can be difficult because of the limited output of masking noise and bone-conduction vibrations.
• This often makes decisions about the potential role of surgery to improve the hearing difficult.
• Behind-the-ear hearing aids are the mainstay of management and involve considerable attention being paid to moulds to allow sufficient gain to be used without feedback.
• Accessory aids, including warning lights, are particularly beneficial for this group.
• Cochlear implants are increasingly likely to be considered in this group especially in those with thresholds worse than 95 dB HL.
• Tinnitus is difficult to mask in this group of patients and reliance is often on counselling.

Further reading

Summerfield, A.Q. and Marshall, D.H. (1995). Cochlear implantation in the UK, 1990–1994. Report by the MRC Institute of Hearing Research in the evaluation of the national cochlear implant programme. HMSO Publications, London.

12 Hearing impairment in infants

Incidence

As in adults, hearing impairment in infants under the age of 3 years can affect one or both ears to a varying degree and be sensorineural, conductive or mixed in type. Because of the difficulties in testing in this age group, prevalence data are difficult to obtain, particularly for the impairments. What is known is the prevalence of children who by the age of 2–3 years have been identified as having an impairment worse than 40 dB HL in their better hearing ear (*Table 12.1*). The overall prevalence is 133 per 100,000 or 1.3 per 1000 live births and by far the majority are sensorineural in type. Taking these figures, the risk of a child having a hearing impairment worse than 40 dB HL is 1 in 750, of whom 56 per cent will have a mild to moderate (40–69 dB HL), 21 per cent a severe (70–94 dB HL) and 23 per cent a profound (≥ 95 dB HL) impairment.

Table 12.1 Prevalence per 100,000 live births of different degrees of hearing impairment overall and for sensorineural impairments only, with 95 per cent confidence intervals

Degree of impairment (dB HL)	Prevalence per 100,000 (95% CI)	
	Overall	Sensorineural only
≥ 40	133 (122–145)	127 (116–139)
≥ 70	59 (52–68)	59 (51–67)
≥ 95	31 (26–37)	31 (26–37)
≥ 40–69	74 (65–83)	68 (61–78)
70–94	28 (23–35)	28 (23–34)

(After Fortnum and Davis, 1997)

Such children are usually identified by a combination of methods including parental concern, by screening and by slow development of speech and language.

Aetiology

Hearing impairments in infants can be categorized as 'congenital', that is present around the time of birth, or 'acquired', that is the hearing is presumed to be normal at birth. Congenital impairments are subdivided into genetic, intra-uterine and perinatal according to when the impairment is likely to have developed. *Table 12.2* lists the main recognized causes,

Table 12.2 More frequent causes of hearing impairment in infants categorized according to type of impairment

Sensorineural:			
	Congenital		
		Genetic	Syndromal, e.g. Turner's
			Non-syndromal
		Intra-uterine	Infection, e.g. rubella
	Perinatal		e.g. hypoxia
	Acquired	Infection	e.g. meningitis
		Other	e.g. trauma
Conductive:			
	Congenital		
		Genetic	Syndromal, e.g. Treacher Collins
			Non-syndromal, e.g. osteogenesis imperfecta
	Acquired	Inflammation	Otitis media

some aspects of which are discussed below. In a high proportion of those with a sensorineural impairment the aetiology is uncertain.

Congenital

Genetically predetermined 'deafness' is easy to suspect if the child has one of the commoner syndromes. These are not listed here but can be read about in longer texts (e.g. Adams, 1997a; Fraser 1976). Those involving obvious cranio-facial abnormalities (e.g. Down's, Crouzon's disease, Treacher Collins, Pierre Robin; Apert's, Klippel-Feil) are more likely to be associated with a conductive impairment. Those involving systemic disorders (e.g. Turner's, Usher's, Alport's) are more likely to have a sensorineural impairment. It is also easy to suspect an inherited disorder in parents that have been hearing impaired since childhood. What are more difficult to suspect and diagnose are spontaneous genetic mutations. Genetic counselling and screening of 'at risk' mothers during pregnancy for Down's syndrome along with legalized abortion has perhaps reduced the number of genetically determined deaf children in developed countries.

Intra-uterine infection

Hopefully the infective causes of infant deafness which develops during gestation are now less common with childhood vaccination, particularly against rubella (German measles). Syphilis can be identified by maternal screen-ing. The foetus may also be infected by cytomegalovirus or toxoplasmosis and this is usually subclinical when the child is born.

Perinatal

The perinatal period is defined as the first 48 hours after birth. In children born prematurely, multiple factors can interplay to cause a hearing impairment. There is the reason for the immaturity, the hypoxia that often goes with premature birth, the infant's susceptibility to infection and the antibiotics given to treat this.

Acquired sensorineural impairments

Bacterial meningitis

This is the commonest cause of acquired sensorineural impairments, about 10 per cent of children with bacterial meningitis becoming impaired with about a quarter of these having a profound deafness (Fortnum and Davis, 1993). Hence screening of hearing should be mandatory in such children once they have recovered. Fortunately, viral meningitis does not affect the hearing.

Other causes

Mumps and measles are well-recognized causes of a sensorineural impairment. The problem is that often these infections are subclinical and many cases are diagnosed by conjecture rather than by antibody assay.

Acquired conductive impairments

Otitis media with effusion

This condition is discussed elsewhere (Chapter 13). Unfortunately, because of its incidence of around 50 per cent at some time during the first 2 years of life, otitis media with effusion is often considered to be the sole cause of an impairment when it is in fact additive to a pre-existing sensorineural impairment. Children with cranio-facial abnormalities, such as occur with Down's syndrome, are also more likely to suffer from otitis media than normal children.

Detection of hearing-impaired infants

It would seem sensible that infants with severe or poorer hearing should be detected as early as possible because amplification with hearing aids or cochlear implants is effective in aiding speech and language development. The desire for early intervention is because the auditory pathways mature and become less adaptable with age. Unless stimulated the intricate interconnecting auditory pathways do not develop and become unable to do so at a later date. This has become evident with cochlear implants where the age of implantation of prelingually deaf children is crucial to success. It is for this reason that most developed countries have instituted some form of screening to detect hearing-impaired infants. The method varies from country to country and within countries from region to region.

Because of the low incidence of hearing impairment, screening has to be closely monitored to ensure that not only are the majority of impaired children detected but also that the number of children falsely labelled as impaired is kept to a minimum. This means that the screening technique has to be both highly sensitive and specific. To take an example, if the sensitivity and specificity of a test are both 90 per cent and the test is used for universal screening where the prevalence of hearing impairment is 1 in 1000, the number of children incorrectly identified as impaired will greatly outnumber the children that are impaired. Thus, in this example the one impaired child in the 1000 will have a 90 per cent chance of being identified. Of the 999 non-impaired children, 10 per cent (i.e. 99.9) will be incorrectly labelled as impaired because the specificity is 90 per cent.

Universal (i.e. total) screening

At 6–12 months

In the UK, health visitors routinely visit the home when the child is between 6 and 12 months of age to check their general development. At this visit the hearing is checked by distraction testing (see below). The practical problem with this approach is that: (a) about 20 per cent of children are never screened because they are not at home; and (b) unless health visitors are well and repeatedly trained distraction testing has a sensitivity in the region of 40 per cent. There is also a tendency for them to incorrectly reassure the parents that any suspicions they may have regarding the child's hearing are unfounded.

Neonatal

Now that semi-automated screening techniques (e.g. oto-acoustic emissions, auditory brain stem responses) are available which have a sensitivity and specificity of around 90 per cent in detecting hearing impairment, some suggest that all children should be screened before discharge from hospital. Apart from the logistical and cost problems with this approach: (a) not all children are born in hospital; and (b) such screening by nature of its timing will not identify those with an acquired impairment, which accounts for around 20 per cent of this hearing-impaired population. Universal neonatal screening has thus to be supplemented by some other screening later on.

Targeted screening

Neonatal

Targeted neonatal screening is where children at particular risk of having a congenital hearing impairment are tested before they leave hospital. Different criteria can be used to construct an 'at risk' register but the easiest to use is: (1) all children with syndromes; (2) all with a family history of hearing impairment; and (3) all children that have been in special care baby units (SCBU). As compared with universal screening this approach reduces the number of children being screened to 10 per cent but in theory should still identify 50 per cent of

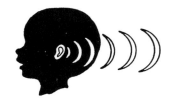

"Can your baby hear you?"

Here is a checklist of some of the general signs you can look for in your baby's first year:-   YES/NO

Shortly after birth
Your baby should be startled by a sudden loud noise such as a hand clap or a door slamming and should blink or open his eyes widely to such sounds.

By 1 Month
Your baby should be beginning to notice sudden prolonged sounds like the noise of a vacuum cleaner and he should pause and listen to them when they begin.

By 4 Months
He should quieten or smile to the sound of your voice even when he cannot see you. He may also turn his head or eyes toward you if you come up from behind and speak to him from the side.

By 7 Months
He should turn immediately to your voice across the room or to very quiet noises made on each side if he is not too occupied with other things.

By 9 Months
He should listen attentively to familiar everyday sounds and search for very quiet sounds made out of sight. He should also show pleasure in babbling loudly and tunefully.

By 12 Months
He should show some response to his own name and to other familiar words. He may also respond when you say 'no' and 'bye bye' even when he cannot see any accompanying gesture.

> Your health visitor will perform a routine hearing screening test on your baby between six and eight months of age. She will be able to help and advise you at any time before or after this test if you are concerned about your baby and his development. If you suspect that your baby is not hearing normally, either because you cannot answer yes to the items above or for some other reason, then seek advice from your health visitor.

Figure 12.1 The Hints for Parents 'Can your baby hear you? form [from *Paediatric Otolaryngology*, Vol. 6, Scott-Brown's Otolaryngology, 6th Edition. Butterworth-Heinemann, Oxford (1997)]

the impaired population. This compares with the 80 per cent of the hearing-impaired population that would be identified by universal neonatal screening.

Stimulated referral

Many parents become suspicious that their infant might be hard of hearing or slow to develop speech but are unwilling to seek advice for many reasons including that they do not want their suspicions to be confirmed. To overcome this and to stimulate parents who might not otherwise have thought about it, check lists such as 'Can your baby hear you?' (*Figure 12.1*) can be issued at the time of the health visitor assessment and be available at other contact points. An alternative is to send out questionnaires to parents.

Spontaneous referral

In most developing countries this is the sole means of identification and in developed countries it is still the means of referral of a high proportion of children including those that missed health visitor screening, those that falsely passed this screen and those with an acquired impairment. The type of person from whom advice is sought varies. It could be from a primary care physician, a community health officer or a health visitor. All should take parental concern seriously and arrange for the hearing to be assessed by a method other than distraction testing.

Assessment of hearing

Various techniques are available, the choice of which to use depending upon availability, the age of the infant, whether there are other developmental abnormalities and whether it is being used as a screening technique or to determine frequency-specific thresholds (*Table 12.3*). The latter are essential for aiding. Techniques can also be categorized as to whether they need a trained technician or not. In this age group otitis media with effusion is common, and may be the sole cause of an impairment or be additive to a sensorineural impairment. Tympanometry (see p. 138) should thus be carried out in all that fail a screening test.

Distraction testing

This is the classical screening method used by health visitors in the UK for infants older than 6 months that can sit upright on their mother's knee. The test is usually carried out in a quiet room with two testers. The child sits on the mother's lap and its attention is held by a tester playing with toys on a table in front of the child. The other tester is behind the mother to one side out of vision of the child and shakes a rattle, hits a tea cup, etc. A hearing child should turn in response to the sound. More frequency-specific threshold information can be obtained using a sound-generating box which produces warble tones. False-positive responses are common and can be mistakenly considered to be normal hearing.

Table 12.3 Audiometric techniques suitable for infants

Technique	Age (months)	Test type	
		Screen	Threshold
Distraction testing	6–24	✔	✔
VRA	6+		✔
Conditioned (play)	24+		✔
ABR	0+	✔	✔
OAE	0+	✔	
ARC	0+	✔	

VRA = visual reinforced audiometry; ABR = auditory brain stem response; OAE = oto-acoustic emissions; ARC = auditory response cradle

Visual reinforced audiometry

This is carried out in a sound-proofed room with the mother and first tester in the same position as for distraction testing. Another tester presents pure tones at calibrated loudness levels, free-field via a loudspeaker in front of the child or through one of two loudspeakers, one on either side. A correct turning of the infant to the relevant loudspeaker is rewarded (reinforced) by flashing the eyes of a toy on the loudspeaker.

Conditioned (play) audiometry

This can be carried out free-field or with headphones and is essentially pure tone audiometry but with the infant carrying out a task, such as putting a peg in a hole or a brick on a stack, rather than raising their hand when they hear a tone.

Speech audiometry

This technique is obviously not applicable to infants who do not have language comprehension. The words used are available as toys or as drawings and the infant's task is to pick up or point to the relevant article when instructed to 'show me the ___'. The speech can be presented free-field or via headphones at various sound levels.

Auditory brain stem (ABR)

The electrical activity in the auditory nerve and brain stem in response to clicks can be recorded by scalp electrodes (see Appendix VII). Simplified, highly automated instruments are available which do not require the tracings to be evaluated and hence can be used by partly trained technicians. The results are not frequency specific but can be recorded without sedation in newborn infants.

Oto-acoustic emissions (OAE)

Highly automated instruments to measure oto-acoustic emissions (see Appendix VIII) are now available which print out the results. This technique is quick and easy to administer – it only requires an ear probe and can be done on a sleeping infant. As it will detect impairments of 25 dB HL or poorer there is a high pick-up rate of otitis media with effusion.

Auditory response cradle

This records a child's movement in response to sound but the technique has been superseded by ABR and OAE.

Management

Hearing aids

Personal hearing aid requirements are no different in children than in adults with the same degree of impairment (Chapter 11). Binaural fitting is usually attempted, but what is different are the technical aspects of fitting and the use of group communication hearing devices for education.

Fitting problems

In an infant holding a behind-the-ear aid in place and preventing it being pulled off can, to some extent, be overcome with sticky tapes and headbands. An alternative is to use a body-worn aid with the connecting wire threaded through the clothes.

Because of the uncertainty there always is in

assessing the thresholds, the most suitable frequency response of the aid and the appropriate gain are often a matter of conjecture rather than measurement. Equally, adjustment of the aid to the correct volume cannot be accurately indicated by a young child. Loudness discomfort has to be avoided as this will make the child intolerant of the aid but the volume has to be sufficiently loud to gain benefit. Parents and teachers also have to check daily whether the aid is functioning as breakdown problems are frequent because of the excess trauma the aids often receive in this age group.

Children have to be reviewed regularly as they get older in an audiology department with suitably trained staff, as aid modifications can be made as the child becomes more able to respond to testing. Equally, frequent changes of ear mould (about once a year) are necessary because of the growth of the pinna and ear canal.

Educational aids

Various aids are available for teaching impaired children when they are in groups or singly. Their main advantage is that they increase the signal-to-noise ratio by selectively picking up the teacher's voice. The teacher wears a microphone/transmitter from which their voice is heard by the child directly by cabling, FM radio, infra-red or a loop system. Except for the loop system, the child requires a personal aid with a receiving socket which uses the 'T' position.

Bone-anchored hearing aids

In those without a pinna to hold an ear mould, bone-conduction aiding is the only option. This is often the case in Treacher Collins syndrome and bilateral congenital atresia. Surgery to create a pinna and canal is a potential option but can be technically difficult and usually requires several operations. It is also usually not embarked upon until the child is older. Now that titanium pegs can be used to anchor plastic ear prostheses and bone-anchored hearing aids (BAHA; see p. 104) these are increasingly the favoured option. As it is generally held that because of the thinness of the skull a peg for an aid should not be inserted

until a child is 2–3 years old, aiding before this is with conventional bone-conduction aids. In those with cranio-facial abnormalities the skull can be particularly thin and the sigmoid sinus and middle cranial fossae may be in abnormal positions. Special care has thus to be taken in such cases when choosing the site for implantation. Pegs for ear prostheses are usually inserted about the time the child goes to secondary school.

Cochlear implants

It is generally accepted that most children with acquired profound or total deafness following meningitis or a head injury will benefit quickly from a cochlear implant. Following meningitis, many argue that this should be done sooner rather than later because of the risk of intra-cochlear ossification which would prevent an electrode being inserted.

Whether prelingually deafened children should be implanted remains controversial. Deaf parents with congenitally deaf children have argued against this because they wish to maintain the culture of sign language. Non-deaf parents do not agree. Obviously it is essential that the hearing thresholds are shown to be virtually absent before implantation, usually by electrocochleography. Implantation is usually carried out about 2 years of age. Unfortunately, because of loss of neural plasticity, the older the child the poorer the results. It is not thought beneficial to implant prelingually deaf children that have not benefited from conventional aids over the age of about 10 years. The prelingually deaf require considerably more rehabilitation and for a longer period of time than those with an acquired impairment.

Speech

The first thing that has to be decided between the parents and their advisers is what method of communication should be taught. The main determinants of this are the amount of residual hearing, whether the parents themselves use sign language and what facilities are available.

In general the aim is to integrate hearing-impaired children into the general community. Hence the development of speech (oralism) and its comprehension (auralism) are usually aimed for. Many unfortunately do not achieve this to a level where they can be understood outside their own group and prefer to communicate with each other by signing. This is difficult to avoid and in the totally deaf often leads to the sole use of signing. The introduction of cochlear implants and their greater success in teaching children to communicate aurally (albeit with a greater educational input) is likely to reduce the proportion of children that sign.

Teaching

The facilities for teaching hearing-impaired children vary from country to country, and there is still often a substantial voluntary element to this. It is just as important to pay attention to the home environment because a child has to communicate as much there if not more than at school. In the UK, preschool tuition is by peripatetic teachers of the deaf. Ideally they should be instructing the parents how to teach the child to speak and to understand speech with their aids as much as teaching the child themselves. Ensuring that the parents know how to check the aid is also important.

Once a child has reached school age, several options are available. They can be taught in a normal classroom with support from teachers of the deaf, taught in part or all the time in special classes in normal schools, or taught in schools for the deaf.

■ Conclusions

- The prevalence of hearing impairments worse than 40 dB HL in the better ear in infants is 1.3 per 1000 live births, the majority being sensorineural in type.
- The aim is to identify these children as early as possible so that amplification can be provided to aid speech and language development.
- The older a child is when provided with effective amplification, the less able they are to benefit because of loss of neural plasticity of the auditory pathways.
- Cochlear implantation is likely to be increasingly used in infants that do not benefit from conventional hearing aids.
- Screening is advocated to lessen the age at which impaired infants are detected. The method used varies between regions and is determined by historical factors, availability of trained staff and cost.
- Screening can be carried out in the neonatal period or at 6–9 months of age.
- Targeted neonatal screening of 'at risk' children (family history of deafness, cranio-facial abnormalities and management in a special care baby unit) by evoked oto-acoustic emission or auditory brain stem response can in theory detect 50 per cent of impaired infants.

- Universal neonatal screening by such methods could be more cost-effective but has to be supplemented by another screening at 6–9 months to identify those with an acquired impairment.
- Even though the specificity of neonatal screening techniques is around 90 per cent, because of the low prevalence of hearing impairments, many normal hearing children will fail such a screen. This requires careful counselling of the parents and a system whereby the child is more fully assessed audiometrically as soon as possible.
- In the UK, universal (total) screening is currently carried out by distraction testing by health visitors at 6–9 months of age.
- Such distraction testing fails to detect a large proportion of impaired children for many reasons. One of these is the poor sensitivity of the test as usually performed.
- At this age visual response audiometry is more reliable but is not suitable for universal screening because of the time and skills involved.
- In both infants and children, otitis media with effusion is a commoner cause of an impairment than a sensorineural problem. Hence those with an impairment require tympanometry in addition to rule out otitis media with effusion.

• Binaural hearing aids are provided as early as possible but in young children there is the additional problem of deciding the most appropriate gain and frequency response, as well as keeping the aids working and in place.

• Regular review by experienced staff to update the aiding system and assess benefit from aiding is essential.

• In all, speech training and educational support is essential.

Further reading

Adams, D.A. (1997a). The causes of deafness. In *Paediatric Otolaryngology*, Vol. 6, Chap. 4, Scott-Brown's Otolaryngology. Butterworth-Heinemann, Oxford.

Adams, D.A. (1997b). Management of the hearing impaired child. In *Paediatric Otolaryngology*, Vol. 6, Chap. 10, Scott-Brown's Otolaryngology. Butterworth-Heinemann, Oxford.

Davis, A., Bamford, J., Wilson, I., Ramkalavan, T., Forshaw, M. and Wright, S. (1997). A critical review of the role of neonatal screening in the detection of congenital hearing impairment. Report submitted to the UK Department of Health.

Fortnum, H. and Davis, A. (1997). Epidemiology of permanent childhood hearing impairment in the Trent region, 1985–93. *British Journal of Audiology* (in press).

Fraser, G.R. (1976). *The Causes of Profound Deafness in Children*. Baillière Tindall, London.

Gibbin, K.P. (1997). Cochlear implantation in children. In *Paediatric Otolaryngology*, Vol. 6, Chap. 11, Scott-Brown's Otolaryngology. Butterworth-Heinemann, Oxford.

McCormick, B. (1997). Screening and surveillance for hearing impairment in pre-school children. In *Paediatric Otolaryngology*, Vol. 6, Chap. 6, Scott-Brown's Otolaryngology. Butterworth-Heinemann, Oxford.

13 Hearing impairment in children: Otitis media with effusion

In most developed countries, children with a congenital sensorineural hearing impairment will have been identified by the age of 3 years (see Chapter 12). Though otitis media is not infrequent before the age of 3, above that age children that develop hearing problems 'de nouveau' are most likely to have otitis media with effusion (OME). The only other acquired condition is meningitis which is thankfully uncommon and should be readily identifiable (see p. 128). This chapter is about the diagnosis, assessment and management of children with otitis media with effusion, though the possibility of other diagnoses must not be forgotten.

Otitis media with effusion

Otitis media with effusion is one end of a spectrum of pathology that affects the middle ear cleft in infants and children, the other end being acute otitis media (AOM). Essentially the condition is one involving the mucosal lining of the middle ear and Eustachian tube which results in poor aeration of the middle ear. Oxygen is absorbed which results in negative middle ear pressure and there is subsequent retention of middle ear mucus. What the initiating factors are is debated, but in any one child it is likely to be multifactorial. In most, infection (mainly viral but also bacterial) in the nasopharynx is likely to contribute to the mucosal oedema of the Eustachian tube and poor functioning of the mucociliary system. Sometimes, but by no means always, the middle ear fluid becomes infected by bacteria, the middle ear becomes grossly inflamed, and the pressure

rises. The eardrum becomes inflamed and bulging at which time otalgia will develop. This stage is usually called acute otitis media. In the majority, the infection will settle within a few days with no sequelae. In some, the tympanic membrane will rupture, with the release of pus and relief of otalgia. In these circumstances the perforation usually heals spontaneously. In the majority the mucosa will recover but sometimes it becomes metaplastic with an increase in the number of goblet cells and subsequent secretions. If this occurs, otitis media with effusion is likely to be present for some time as a sequela. This is the type of ear in which small numbers of bacteria can sometimes be identified.

On the other hand, there are many children with OME that do not have a history of otalgia or AOM, and here bacterial middle ear infection is less likely to have a role. This is more probable in the older (3 years or more) child where the condition is asymptomatic apart from the hearing impairment and the altered behaviour that can accompany this. There is considerable evidence that repeated upper respiratory infection is a dominant factor in the continuation of the condition. Repeated infection is more likely if the child is in close contact with other children such as at play group, at certain times of the year and perhaps if there is adenoid hypertrophy. In children with cranio-facial abnormalities such as those associated with Down's syndrome and cleft palate, OME is understandably more frequent and persistent.

Presentation

The dominant symptom, if any, of OME is a hearing impairment. In most this is mild and because of the episodic nature of the condition is frequently not noticed. Obviously, if a child has a history of otalgia, parents and childminders are more alert than they might otherwise be to the possibility of a hearing impair-

ment. Equally if such adults have experience of looking after several children, such as sibs or grandchildren, a hearing-impaired child is more obvious. Inattention and turning the TV up is not infrequent in normal hearing children, but are common alerters. In different countries, screening of children for hearing impairment is carried out at different ages, but in the UK it is a frequent route of identification of children with OME.

Should the time with a hearing impairment be prolonged, there is the potential that speech and language development may be delayed. Unfortunately, there is a wide variation in the normal development in speech and language and the indicators of impairment are difficult to detect, there being no generally accepted method of clinical assessment. In children that are being educated, as opposed to being minded, a hearing impairment can impede progress. Parents are often naturally worried about this but, again, the level of 'normal' hearing in children is varied. However, no matter how concern is raised about the hearing, it is important always to investigate the possibility of OME.

Diagnosis

There are various methods of diagnosis, as outlined below. This subject is also discussed in Chapter 4.

Otoscopy

The otoscopic findings in OME are varied and often difficult to distinguish from those in a normal situation. Negative middle ear pressure is often suspected by a more horizontal position of the handle of the malleus, a more cone-shaped appearance of the pars tensa or the appearance of a more prominent annular ligament (neo-annular fold). The middle ear fluid may be evident by a subtle change in colour of the pars tensa, from grey to blue, and

the pars tensa itself may become more opaque due to mild inflammation.

Pneumatic otoscopy is advocated by many and, indeed, if the pars tensa is seen to move, middle ear fluid is unlikely. However, the lack of movement is frequently due to lack of a seal of the canal. In experienced observers otoscopy has a sensitivity of around 90 per cent in detecting OME, such figures being calculated by comparing the otoscopic to myringotomy findings. An individual who has achieved such levels is sometimes called a 'validated otoscopist'.

Unfortunately, it is often not possible to visualize the tympanic membrane because of wax. Removal by syringing is possible but sometimes difficult in an anxious child. Under these circumstances tympanometry can be helpful because it can be performed in the presence of wax. Indeed, it could also be argued that tympanometry should be performed irrespective of any otoscopic findings, to improve the sensitivity and specificity of diagnosis.

Tympanometry

The main role of tympanometry in audiology is to detect OME and it does this well because it gives some idea of the middle ear pressure. This is taken from the position of the peak on the tympanometric tracing. The most frequent classification used is that initially proposed by Jerger *et al.* (1974) (*Table 13.1*). The simplest way to categorize tympanograms is into peaked (A and C) and non-peaked (B) graphs. If this is done, the pressure range over which the ear was tested has to be stated. Thus, some hand-held machines only go down to -200 or -300 mmH$_2$O (deca-Pascals, daPa). Most desk tympanometers go down to -300 or -400 mmH$_2$O and some go down to -600 mmH$_2$O. The problem with machines that go down to a small negative pressure is that a flat tympanogram down to -200 mmH$_2$O could well peak at say -300 mmH$_2$O, thus reclassifying a type B as a type C tympanogram.

Many studies (e.g. Finitzo *et al.*, 1992) have looked at the correlation between tympanogram type and the findings at myringotomy under or shortly after a general anaesthetic. This must be considered the 'gold standard' even though, because of the anaesthetic (N$_2$O) and perhaps positive nasopharyngeal pres-

Table 13.1 Classification of tympanograms

	Type	Description
Peaked	A	Between +200 and −99 mmH$_2$O
	C$_1$	Between −100 and −199 mmH$_2$O
	C$_2$	Between −200 and −399 mmH$_2$O
	C$_3$	Between −400 and −600 mmH$_2$O
Non-peaked	B	No observable peak between +200 and −600 mmH$_2$O

(After Jerger *et al.*, 1974)

sure due to ventilation, a certain number that had fluid will become dry. All papers rank the types of tympanograms in the order B, C$_2$, C$_1$ and A with respect to sensitivity in detecting middle ear fluid (*Table 13.2*). Correspondingly, instead of using peaked versus non-peaked to classify the tympanograms, some use B and C$_2$ versus A and C$_1$ tympanograms (*Table 13.2*). Which is used depends on the purposes for which the tympanogram is being performed because increasing the sensitivity of a test inevitably decreases its specificity (see Appendix I).

Table 13.2 Sensitivity and specificity of tympanometry in identifying OME

	Sensitivity	Specificity	PPV	NPV
B versus rest	57	93	96	47
B + C$_2$ versus rest	88	73	66	53
Otoscopy	93	58	84	77

PPV = positive predictive value; NPV = negative predictive value
(After Finitzo *et al.*, 1992)

Assessment of sequelae

Audiometry

It is agreed that if there is concern about a child's hearing then some form of audiometry to assess the hearing is mandatory. There will be a small number of children ($<$ 1 per cent) that do not have OME but have a congenital sensorineural impairment. Also, children with

OME do not necessarily have a material hearing impairment (*Table 13.3* and *Figures 13.1* and *13.2*). The problem is that audiometry is not always available (e.g. in primary care) and in this age group requires special testing skills and time. Some children do not like wearing headphones let alone bone-conduction bands, though the suggestion is that because of the

Table 13.3 Hearing level (pure tone average over 0.5, 1, 2 and 4 kHz) and air–bone gap (average over 0.5, 1 and 2 kHz) in children with OME, evidenced by a type B tympanogram

	% of ears
Hearing level (dB):	
0–19	10
20–39	70
⩾ 40	20
Air–bone gap (dB):	
0–9	1
10–19	6
20–29	20
30–39	23
⩾ 40	40

(MRC Target data)

'space age' this problem is less frequent than formerly. The other main difficulty is maintaining the child's attention, a problem that is overcome to some extent by using game techniques. Distraction testing is discussed elsewhere as a means of testing 6 month to 2 year old children (see p. 131). Visual reinforced audiometry and play audiometry will be discussed again here.

Visual reinforced audiometry

This is done free-field in a sound-proofed room. The child is sat on someone's knee and their attention held by a distractor. Sound is then presented at suprathreshold levels through one of two loudspeakers at a 90 degree angle to attract the attention of the child. The head turn response is recorded by flashing eyes in a toy on top of the speaker. After the child has been conditioned, the free-field thresholds at different frequencies can be determined in the usual manner. The results obviously reflect binaural rather than monaural hearing. Such testing can usually be done from about the age of 6–12 months. In older children the technique can be altered from free-field to headphone sounds.

Play audiometry

Basically the child is taught to perform some simple task such as putting a peg in a hole or a brick on a stack in response to a sound. This method has the advantage of requiring only one tester and again can be done free-field or with headphones. Children usually have to be two and a half years old to learn the game.

Relation of tympanogram type to hearing

Because audiometry can be time-consuming, it would be helpful if tympanometry could predict which child did not have OME associated with a hearing impairment. Several

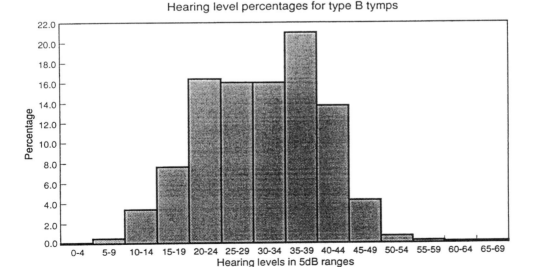

Figure 13.1 Histogram of hearing level (pure tone average over 0.5, 1, 2 and 4 kHz) in children's ears with OME, evidenced by a type B tympanogram (MRC Target data)

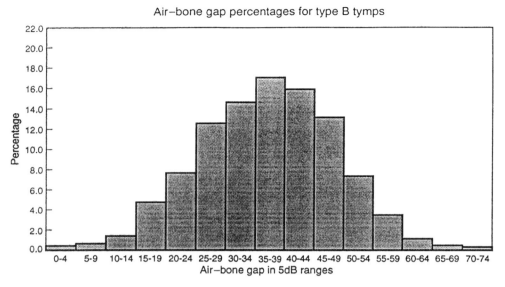

Figure 13.2 Histogram of air–bone gap (over 0.5, 1 and 2 kHz) in children's ears with OME, evidenced by a type B tympanogram (MRC Target data)

studies have assessed the correlation between the different tympanometry types and hearing (Dempster and McKenzie, 1991; Kazanas and Maw, 1994; MRC Multicentre Target Report, 1998). The last article gives the most detailed analysis to date (*Table 13.4*) and is based on 1446 children aged from 3.5 to 7 years referred for an otolaryngological assessment in clinics in the UK because of suspected OME. The predictive values should thus be applicable to clinics with a similar referral pattern. It can be seen that both a B and combining a B with a C_2 tympanogram have high sensitivities and predictive values in identifying the hearing in the better hearing ear. Which to choose (B

or B and C_2) to identify children that require audiometry necessitates a consideration of the fact that increasing sensitivity is achieved to the detriment of specificity.

Speech and language

Unfortunately, except in the grossest cases which usually occur in the multiply handicapped child, abnormalities of speech and language due to mild or moderate hearing impairment are difficult to detect clinically. The rate of development varies enormously especially in the early stages between 1 and 3

Table 13.4 Correlation between tympanometry type and hearing in OME

| | | | | | Pure tone average (dB HL) | | | | Air–bone gap ABG ⩾ 10 | |
| | ⩾ 15 | | ⩾ 20 | | ⩾ 25 | | ⩾ 30 | | | |
	B	B + C_2	B	B + C_2	B	B + C_2	B	B + C_2	B	B + C_2
Sensitivity	81	93	87	97	93	98	96	99	80	93
Specificity	82	63	75	51	59	37	49	31	80	62
PPV	92	87	84	74	61	52	42	35	93	90

PPV = positive predictive value
(MRC Multicentre Target Report, 1998)

years of age and, apart from hearing, is dependent on many other factors, including how much interaction there is with adults and other children in conversation. Various tests have been developed that are applicable to different age groups, but the 'normal' values have a large range and thus such tests are not generally used.

Learning and cognition

It seems reasonable to postulate that a hearing-impaired child is likely to learn and become knowledgeable less quickly than normal. It is not unusual for parents to be concerned about a child's lack of progress at school and be worried about hearing as a cause. If an impairment is present in the better ear and has been documented to be persistent then it cannot be excluded as a contributor though it could be just that the child is a slow learner at that specific time in their life.

Behaviour

A child's behaviour is dependent on their personality and their interaction with a particular environment. With illness this can change with them being tired, lethargic, irritable, fractious, etc. It would seem reasonable that a child with an upper respiratory tract infection with secondary otalgia and middle ear fluid will be 'different' from their normal selves. Whether a child that is otherwise 'normal', apart from a hearing impairment due to OME, will behave differently is not known.

Natural history of OME

Before deciding on management, it is helpful to know what the natural history of the untreated condition is and what are the outcomes.

Several studies have followed up children over various age ranges to ascertain the incidence of OME and chart its natural history. The results vary greatly. Unfortunately, different methods of diagnosing OME have been used which make meta-analysis difficult, but *Figure 13.3* shows the prevalence, with 95 per cent confidence intervals, of various studies (Zielhuis *et al.*, 1990). The prevalence falls off after the age of 5 years. Before that the prevalence is in the region of 15 per cent with the suggestion of a binaural peak at 2.5 and 5 years which can be interpreted as the age at which children start attending nursery and primary schools, respectively. There is certainly considerable evidence that the incidence is higher in children attending play groups, day care, etc., where there is multiple contact with other children.

There is a suggestion that boys are more frequently affected than girls and that the dura-

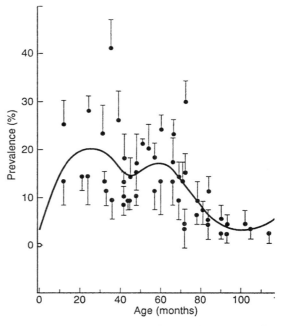

Figure 13.3 Combined results of selected studies on the prevalence of OME with 95 per cent confidence levels (after Zielhuis *et al.*, 1990)

tion of the effusion is longer in boys (Daly, 1991). This is in keeping with the greater susceptibility of boys to infective conditions.

The incidence in the Northern hemisphere is season dependent with the highest incidence in the winter, falling off in the summer and building up again in the autumn (*Table 13.5*). Whether this is really an effect of climate such as temperature or humidity rather than being a surrogate for being indoors and in closer contact with others in the 'bad' season is not known. It has been suggested that OME is uncommon in some racial groups in some countries (e.g. South Africa, Hong Kong) and, if confirmed, this gives a considerable opportunity to tease out the risk factors. What the other risk factors are for the development of OME are controversial, it being essential that all the relevant factors are looked at in a multifactorial manner. Unfortunately, it seems that no study of this type has yet been carried out.

Once OME has developed in one or both

Table 13.5 Seasonal prevalence of OME in 4 year old children where OME is defined from a $B + C_2$ tympanogram

Feb	May	Aug	Nov	Feb
43	35	33	38	50

(After Tos *et al.*, 1982)

ears, the majority of cases resolve in 6–12 weeks. There are some in whom the condition persists and in those that resolve some will get recurrent episodes. As the sequelae of OME are more likely to be related to the duration of OME rather than anything else, the clinical objective is to try and identify those that have persistent OME and those that have frequent OME. This is achieved by a period of watchful waiting. Thus if a child has OME, they are reviewed 3 months later, and if the condition is still present they fall into the group of having persistent or recurrent OME.

Sequelae/outcomes

Pathological changes

Permanent retraction of areas of the pars tensa and pars flaccida are not uncommon in ears that have had OME. Histologically, there can be loss of the fibrous layer in the area of retracted pars tensa and it can become adherent to the long process of the incus and/or promontory. In a few cases, progressive necrosis of the long process of the incus can occur. In a very few others the retraction can be out of vision in the attic or posterior middle ear which may lead to the retention of squamous debris and the development of a cholesteatoma.

The prevalence of such sequelae is uncertain, particularly as the condition is a continuing dynamic process (Tos *et al.*, 1987). Thus, tympanosclerotic patches can resolve or continue to develop and retracted areas can progress to cholesteatoma. Overall, about 50 per cent of ears that have had OME are scarred,

tympanosclerotic, thin or retracted. Less than 1 per cent develop a cholesteatoma. There is minimal if any evidence that management, particularly with ventilation tubes, affects the incidence of these sequelae. Indeed this could increase the prevalence of pars tensa abnormalities particularly by the development of chronic perforations in about 5 per cent of ears at the site of the extruded ventilation tube.

Speech and language

It is accepted that children with a congenital severe or profound impairment are retarded in their development of speech and language. At what age and for how long a mild to moderate impairment has to be present in OME for speech and language to be affected is not known but is obviously dependent on other factors. As discussed earlier, there is no generally accepted standardized test available for any age group, mainly because the assessment of speech and language has many different aspects. Because of the temporary nature of the impairment in OME, it is also thought that the majority of children will catch up fairly quickly. Though there is no evidence to support it, it is considered that a bilateral hearing impairment of 6 months' duration is unlikely to lead to any permanent loss of speech and language deficit at any age.

Behaviour/learning/quality of life

Whilst poor behaviour, slower learning and an overall reduced quality of life for both the child and their carers seems likely during the time that OME is present, whether the effect is a long term one is unproven. Studies are on small numbers, which makes it difficult to separate out the effect of OME from the other factors that affect behaviour, learning and quality of life such as home background and maternal input.

Management

Primary management

In many countries the initial diagnosis will be made by non-specialists with no direct access to tympanometry or audiometry.

After diagnosis the parents should be told that, although their child has 'glue ear' (OME), in the vast majority of instances the hearing impairment is mild, and that natural resolution is the norm over a few weeks or months with no permanent sequelae. Such reassurance is both truthful and helps counteract any previous misconceptions that there may well have been because of parent gossip. If a child is prone to recurrent episodes of otalgia with presumed AOM, prophylactic antibodies do not really have a role (Appelman *et al.*, 1991; Casselbrant *et al.*, 1992). Otherwise, there is no need to consider any medication. Various medications such as nasal decongestants, mucolytics, antihistamines, nasal steroids and antibodies have all been suggested as potential therapies. Randomized controlled trials have shown these to have only a minor effect, if any, for a short period of time. Many clinicians use them but recognize that any effect is likely to be a placebo one.

In theory, auto-inflation should be effective. The problem is that few children can carry out a standard Valsalva manoeuvre. An alternative is to blow up balloons via the nose using a plastic nose-piece (Otovent). A surprising number of children (and their parents) cannot blow up a balloon with their mouth, let alone their nose, but it is certainly worth attempting in the older child.

The parents and those involved with looking after the child should of course modify their behaviour in communicating with them. Ensuring that speech-reading is practical is perhaps the most important element in this.

If a child is considered after a 3 month follow-up period still to have bilateral OME then referral for audiometric assessment and management is indicated. Otherwise, a watchful eye should be kept on the child for recurrence.

Secondary management

The first task on receiving such a referral is to confirm the diagnosis of OME by otoscopy and tympanometry. Having done that a formal audiometric assessment is important as this is the only way of quantifying the degree of hearing impairment in the better hearing ear. What level of pure tone average constitutes an impairment in this age group is not agreed and depends considerably on how reliable the audiometric results are considered to be. In general, the simplest audiometric method should be used (see above). A material impairment is unlikely if the four frequency air-conduction average is better than 20 dB HL. If this was indeed the case in the better ear, most secondary centres would reassure the parents that, although their child may have OME, the impairment associated with it is minor, and the child would be referred back to primary care. This is likely to be the situation in at least four out of five children referred (MRC Target data). In those with an impairment in their better ear, a further watchful waiting period of at least 3 months is advocated, as about 50 per cent of children followed up at this stage will have sufficient resolution of their OME not to have a hearing impairment in their better ear (MRC Target data). Such resolution also appears to occur irrespective of the duration of the history before referral. During this watchful waiting period, medical management is an option if it is felt that something 'active' needs to be done and is the same as discussed under primary management. In children whose impairment persists, most would consider surgery at this stage.

Surgical options

Myringotomy, aspiration of fluid and the insertion of ventilation tubes (grommets) in the anterior tympanic membrane is the most effective option. Various designs of ventilation tubes in different materials are available. Most surgeons have their favourite but, in general, they can be classified as short or long term based on how long on average they remain in the tympanic membrane before being spontaneously extruded. Short term tubes stay in position for 6 months to a year, and long term ones up to two years, the design difference being how large the flange is that is inserted on the middle ear side. The main problem with ventilation tubes is the 30 per cent incidence of secondary infection. Apart from the associated otorrhoea, infection can block the vent, encourage its extrusion and/or be associated with a permanent small perforation. It is for these reasons that long term ventilation tubes are inadvisable for OME, certainly in the first instance.

Controlled clinical trials (Maw and Herod, 1986; Dempster *et al.*, 1993; Effective Health Care Bulletin No.4, 1992) of ventilation tubes against no surgery have shown that the hearing is materially improved over 6–12 months. By that time the condition in the non-treated ear will usually have resolved. After the insertion of ventilation tubes the child should be

reassessed audiometrically every 3 months and, should the impairment recur (perhaps due to a blocked or extruded vent), then reinsertion may be warranted.

Many surgeons advocate adenoidectomy at the time of ventilation tube insertion. Adenoidectomy on its own is ineffective in about 50 per cent of ears, but it does increase the benefit to hearing in about 50 per cent of ears that have a ventilation tube inserted, particularly in the long term. Unfortunately, it is not possible to predict which children would particularly benefit. Adenoidectomy is potentially a more serious operation than inserting ventilation tubes in that troublesome bleeding sometimes occurs and there is the rare problem of hypernasality and speech defects. Ventilation tubes can be inserted as a day case, but adenoidectomy is more problematical and often merits admission overnight. Hence, adenoidectomy is often reserved for persistent cases that require ventilation tubes to be reinserted.

In children, ventilation tubes are usually inserted under an inhalational general anaesthetic. This may include nitrous oxide which diffuses into the middle ear. Alternatively the nasopharyngeal pressure may be increased by the pressure of ventilation. In a few cases (about 10 per cent) this will encourage ventilation of the middle ear before the myringotomy is performed, resulting in a 'dry' tap. Under these circumstances, if a hearing impairment is well documented up until the time of surgery, then most would still insert a ventilation tube. On the other hand, if there has been a delay, a 'dry' tap more likely indicates natural resolution of the condition and insertion of a ventilation tube is probably not warranted.

Follow-up after surgery is important for many reasons. First and frequently forgotten is a necessity to check by audiometry that surgery has improved the hearing. This is often the time that a previously unrecognized sensorineural impairment is recognized. If the hearing has not improved or deteriorated, the ventilation tube may be blocked by 'glue' or pus. Alternatively it may have been extruded. These possibilities are looked for otoscopically supplemented by tympanometry. If the tympanogram is flat, the OME has recurred because of a non-functioning tube. If the hearing impairment persists then reinsertion of the ventilation tube will be considered.

A major problem with tubes is infection

which occurs in about 30 per cent of ears. Prophylaxis against this by the use of antibiotic steroid drops at the time of surgery has its advocates, backed up by some randomized controlled trials but not by others. The infection is frequently silent without otalgia because the middle ear pus can drain via the tube. Treat- ment would appear important to prevent extrusion and to decrease the chances of a permanent tympanic membrane perforation occurring. The incidence of this is about 5 per cent. Aural toilet with topical antibiotic steroid drops is usually helpful. Systemic antibiotics are less likely to be beneficial.

■ Conclusions

• The main diagnosis to consider in a child that acquires a hearing impairment is otitis media with effusion (also known as serous otitis media, secretory otitis media, non-purulent otitis media, chronic non-suppurative otitis media or glue ear).
• Otitis media with effusion is one end of a spectrum of otitis medias in childhood. The other end of the spectrum is acute otitis media.
• In a child aged 3 years or older otitis media with effusion is frequently asymptomatic and suspected by parents or a child's teacher because of inattention due to a hearing impairment.
• Diagnosis is by a combination of otoscopy, tympanometry and audiometry.
• A flat tympanogram (type B or C_2) is a sensitive indicator of otitis media with effusion.
• Audiometry with visual response or play is essential to identify those with an associated hearing impairment of a severity that merits follow-up.
• Because of the high rate of spontaneous resolution a period of watchful waiting of 3 months or longer is recommended before considering surgical intervention.

• No medication is of unequivocal value in hastening resolution long term.
• Children with persistent bilateral otitis media and a hearing impairment in their better hearing ear are perhaps at risk from delay in their speech and language development.
• Ventilation tubes (grommets) are of proven value in improving the hearing. By the time they extrude spontaneously the otitis media with effusion will have resolved naturally.
• In some, adenoidectomy has an additive effect in improving the hearing.
• The pathological sequelae of otitis media with effusion include tympanic membrane retraction, tympanosclerosis and chronic otitis media. These appear to be unaffected by the insertion of ventilation tubes.

Further reading

Department of Health and Human Services (1994). Managing otitis media with effusion in young children. *Quick Reference Guide for Clinicians*, **12**.
Effective Health Care Bulletin (1992). The treatment of persistent glue ear in children. *Effective Health Care*, **4**.

14 Tinnitus

Tinnitus is a common symptom and, depending on how it is defined, between 15 and 30 per cent of the adult British population have noises in their ears or head at some time or other (MRC Institute of Hearing Research, 1981 and 1984; General Household Survey, 1983). In the majority of cases the tinnitus is intermittent and of short duration. Of these individuals only one in seven is likely to be troubled 'a great deal or quite a lot' (General Household Study, 1983). Understandably, those with continuous tinnitus are more likely to be troubled, the proportion being one in three. Other data have shown that 0.5 per cent of the adult population have tinnitus which severely affects their ability to lead a normal life (MRC Institute of Hearing Research, 1984).

Most individuals with tinnitus will also have a hearing impairment, even though many of them have not noticed it. Hearing impairments are usually detected by pure tone audiometry but it cannot be assumed that if the thresholds at the standard test frequencies are normal, the hearing is truly normal. Pure tone audiometry only tests a few frequencies and it is quite conceivable that there is a loss in the audiogram which has gone undetected (Sirimanna *et al.*, 1996). Moreover, there may be audiometric abnormalities present which cannot be detected by conventional means (McKee and Stephens, 1992).

It is often considered that tinnitus is more frequently associated with noise-induced hearing loss than with any other type or cause of impairment. Recent studies (MRC Institute of Hearing Research, 1984) would suggest that this is not the case, it is just that noise is the commonest identifiable cause of a sensorineural hearing impairment. Overall, about 50 per cent of those with a substantial ($\geqslant 50$ dB HL) hearing impairment will also have tinnitus, irrespective of its aetiology or whether it is a conductive or a sensorineural impairment. In any age group and social class, the prevalence of tinnitus is directly related to the prevalence of hearing impairment and this is also likely to apply to children. One anomaly that at present cannot be explained is that women of all age groups are more likely to report tinnitus than men.

Tinnitus is often arbitrarily divided into objective and subjective tinnitus. Objective tinnitus is where the clinician can hear the noises that the patient is complaining of by listening to the patient's ear, head or neck. Subjective tinnitus is where only the patient can hear the sounds. The distinction between these two types of tinnitus is sometimes uncertain; for example, is tinnitus caused by oto-acoustic emissions, which can only be 'heard' when amplified, objective or subjective? The way of solving this dilemma is that if a physical cause for the tinnitus is identified, the cause is stated. For example, a vascular bruit is called a vascular bruit and the term 'tinnitus' would be reserved for what was previously known as subjective tinnitus.

Pathophysiology

The aetiology of tinnitus is at present unknown, several theories having been postulated but none proven. Perhaps the most favoured, and certainly the one easiest to give to patients, is that some of the hair cells are mildly damaged and send out a different pattern of signals which the brain then interprets as sounds. In reality there is no reason why the site of the problem should be in the cochlea or auditory nerve. Central tinnitus is likely in patients in whom bilateral tinnitus is relieved by unilateral masking. Why a conductive hearing impairment in the middle ear should give rise to tinnitus is more difficult to explain unless it is because of an associated or coincidental age-related sensorineural impairment that frequently accompanies these conditions.

History

The most important facts to elicit from the patient's history regarding the tinnitus are outlined below.

Does the patient have tinnitus?

Patients that are concerned about their tinnitus usually mention it in the interview. Those that are not troubled frequently omit to mention it until pressed. Because the identification of tinnitus has no diagnostic role, the main reason for enquiring as to its presence is for management. The patient should not be asked 'Do you have tinnitus?', as many symptoms can come under this label such as ear popping or earache. Rather they should be asked if they have any noises or buzzing in the ears or head.

What does it sound like?

It is important to find out what the patient actually hears to confirm that he has tinnitus and to help to exclude the rare patient who hears voices or 'enemy machinery'. Such patients are usually considered to have a major psychiatric disorder rather than a telepathic trait. A subgroup actually have tinnitus but translate it into music or singing.

The majority complain of sounds that buzz or hiss but if the sound pulsates a vascular cause should be suspected and the clinical examination should be directed towards this. Equally if the tinnitus is of a clicking nature, a pharyngeal or tympanic muscle twitch should be suspected. It is not unusual for patients to have more than one tinnitus sound so, for example, they might have a constant hiss, in addition to which they might intermittently have a ringing sound.

Where are the sounds heard?

For management purposes, it is relevant to ask where the sounds are mainly heard. In essence the tinnitus can be in only one ear, mainly one ear, equally in both ears or 'in the head'.

Are the sounds continuously or intermittently present?

It is important to know whether the tinnitus is intermittently or continuously present as this usually reflects the amount of trouble the patient has, if any. It is sometimes surprisingly difficult to distinguish between the two types. Tinnitus may be continuously present but only noticed when the patient thinks about it or when it is quiet. Such a patient has continuous tinnitus but only intermittently notices it. Individuals with intermittent tinnitus will have definite spells when the tinnitus is not present.

How much distress does the tinnitus cause?

Tinnitus in the vast majority of cases causes little distress. In such patients an explanation as to its likely cause and reassurance that its presence is not a predictor of progressive deafness or increasing tinnitus is probably all that is necessary. A lesser number are sometimes disturbed, often when they are relatively inactive such as in the evening, and may require some form of management in addition to reassurance. Even fewer are seriously disturbed and require considerable time and effort in their management. Rather surprisingly, it is not usually the relative loudness of the tinnitus that matters but whether the patient can learn to live with it. When measurements are made of the relative loudness of tinnitus, the levels are only about 5–15 dB above the patient's worst pure tone threshold. To many this might appear an insignificant amount of noise and engender disinterest. However, it is easy for everyone to think of situations where sounds can be irritating. For example, during a concert the rustle of a sweet paper can produce distress totally out of proportion to its loudness. This is an example where it is not the loudness of the sound that matters but the psychological reaction to it. In a patient it could be that a sound of 10 dB is actually much louder in comparison with normal because of recruitment. Enquiry can fairly rapidly categorize the patient's degree of distress and in those that are seriously disturbed, attention should also be paid to the patient's personality.

What is the patient's personality?

Most otologists will not have had a psychiatric training, but it should be possible for them to assess the patient's personality. The actual proportions falling into each category depend on the referral pattern to a clinic.

Normal personality

Such individuals are able to cope with their tinnitus most of the time. They constitute by far the majority of individuals with tinnitus and usually only require an explanation of what tinnitus is. In such patients, spending too much time discussing their tinnitus can be counterproductive and cause concern.

Introspective or obsessive personality

Introspective or obsessive patients require more time in counselling. They usually turn up with a written list of questions to ask but with sufficient time for discussion they will usually adjust to their tinnitus.

Depressive personality

Depressed patients are usually easy to recognize. There is a certain hopelessness about their attitude and, if one discusses it with them, they usually have some insight as to the relationship between their tinnitus and their depression. Which came first is a matter for debate but the management is usually antidepressant drugs and psychiatric counselling.

Hysterical

These persons do not usually consider themselves to have any psychological problems. Tinnitus is something the patient has and they will complain: 'why can't the medical profession do something for me?'. Usually several doctors will have been consulted in the past in an attempt to get 'cured' and as each 'cure' fails the patient gets more and more involved with their problems. This type of patient often benefits more from tinnitus masking, as this is an obvious physical aid to wear. Psychiatric treatment and formal counselling are usually strongly resisted because they consider themselves to be normal apart from their 'wretched tinnitus'.

Psychotic

This type of personality should be suspected if the patient is withdrawn and introverted and if the tinnitus sounds bizarre such as 'threatening voices'. Psychiatric management is necessary but it can be difficult to get the patient to agree to this.

Are there any provoking factors?

Noise

There is a subset of patients whose tinnitus is exacerbated by background noise rather than masked by it. So, that when they go into a noisy environment, such as a pub, the noise aggravates their tinnitus rather than masks it. Such patients may also have hyperacusis which is an emotional dislike of noise and require a different management approach (see p. 153).

Drugs

Drugs are often blamed for tinnitus but they are seldom responsible. Salicylates are the most obvious exception but it is unusual for them to be taken in high enough dosages to cause tinnitus except when taken for rheumatoid arthritis. Fortunately, if a drug is responsible, the tinnitus usually disappears once the drug has been withdrawn so it is often worthwhile stopping or changing a patient's prescription on the off-chance that the drug was indeed responsible.

Some consider caffeine in tea and coffee and nicotine in cigarettes, pipes and cigars to be causes, but there is no evidence to support this. Alcohol can make some individuals' tinnitus worse, but helps others.

Clinical examination

Patients with tinnitus should have their ears examined and their hearing assessed in the normal manner. In those with pulsatile or clicking tinnitus, an objective cause will be sought.

Pulsatile sounds

There are several possible causes for a patient hearing a pulsation in the ear, the most common one being that they are actually hearing a normal pulsation. This is particularly likely if they have a conductive hearing impairment, which will attenuate environmental noise and allow body sounds to be more easily heard. If a patient can hear the sounds when they are being examined it can be helpful to see if the sounds are synchronous with the pulse. It is also important to exclude the fairly rare causes for a bruit such as glomus jugulare tumours, developmental vascular anomalies and carotid artery stenosis. The neck, skull and ear can be auscultated and the tympanic membrane observed for a glomus tympanicum. These can sometimes be seen to pulsate. Acoustic impedance is an alternative way to look for the latter conditions, as the compliance will vary in time with the pulse.

Muscle twitches

Muscle twitches of the palate, stapedius and tensor tympani muscles are rare causes of tinnitus. Often they can be suspected due to the clicking nature of the noise. Middle ear muscle twitches will not usually be detected by otoscopy but tympanometry may be of value. Palatal twitching can sometimes be detected by examining the palate, preferably by nasendoscopy. One of the problems of diagnosing muscle twitches is that they may be only intermittently present and the clinician has to be fortunate enough to be present when the patient has a twitch. Botulinum toxin injection into the palate is reported to be of benefit (Saeed and Brookes, 1993). Division of the stapedius and tensor tympani muscle would appear to be a simple means of treatment but the results can be disappointing.

Audiometric assessment of tinnitus

Audiometric assessment of a patient with tinnitus starts with standard pure tone audiometry to identify whether an impairment is present and to classify its type. In patients with normal thresholds, testing at non-standard frequencies such as 3 and 6 kHz may identify dips in the audiogram. In those with abnormal thresholds, management is along routine lines, including the investigation of those with asymmetric sensorineural thresholds to exclude retrocochlear pathology.

Many specific tinnitus tests have been proposed but, as they have little diagnostic value and do not help in management, they are not routinely carried out in most clinics. In some clinics they are considered helpful in reassuring the patient that they are being investigated and their symptoms are being taken seriously. Obviously testing is only possible in patients whose tinnitus is present at the time and is thus mainly used in those with troublesome, continuous tinnitus. Testing is used to describe the frequency spectrum and the loudness of a patient's tinnitus, and this is done by *matching* techniques. *Masking* techniques are now seldom used as these are considered less reliable and not of interest in themselves as total masking of a patient's tinnitus is not what is aimed for in the majority of patients (see p. 152).

Matching techniques

An attempt can be made to assess the frequency spectrum of the tinnitus by presenting pure tones to the patient and asking them which tone is nearest in pitch to their tinnitus. There are several problems with this. In most patients the tinnitus is not tonal or even broadband. Most patients find pitch matching difficult and correspondingly there is considerable test/retest variation, so much so that it has been suggested that matching techniques ought to be repeated seven times to improve the reliability of results (Tyler and Conrad-Armes, 1982). Errors also arise because the tinnitus is often above the highest frequency that can be presented for matching. Frequency matching, therefore, can only be a rough guide to the pitch of the tinnitus.

Matching techniques have also been used to assess the relative loudness of the tinnitus. Once a tone on the audiometer has been chosen as the one most similar in pitch to the tinnitus, this may be presented and the intensity adjusted until a loudness match is obtained. Again there are many problems. Which ear should the tone be presented to? There may be recruitment. The chosen tone may not be correct.

Management

By the time the clinician comes to management, patients can usually be ascribed to one of four categories:

(1) Hearing impaired; tinnitus identified only on enquiry.
(2) Hearing impaired; tinnitus mentioned but minor concern.
(3) Tinnitus dominant symptom; first specialist consultation.
(4) Tinnitus dominant symptom; previous specialist opinion.

In all, the main thrust in management is to reduce the concern the patient might have regarding the tinnitus and suggest management appropriate to their degree of concern.

Hearing impaired; tinnitus identified only on enquiry

Here, the management is of the hearing impairment along with a reassurance that 50 per cent of patients with a similar hearing impairment will have tinnitus, that is not caused by a tumour or brain disease and in the vast majority it is not a problem. What has to be avoided in such patients is negative counselling. This can easily be given by suggesting that there are people who are seriously upset by their tinnitus, that it is a lifelong problem that never goes away, that self-help groups are available and that there is considerable advisory literature on the condition.

Hearing impaired; tinnitus mentioned but minor concern

Management is primarily of the hearing impairment, with provision of an aid to the side with the most dominant tinnitus. It should be explained that the use of the aid will almost certainly make the tinnitus less obvious because of the introduction of background noise. This should occur even with a monaural aid and tinnitus 'in the head'.

Positive counselling

These patients should receive positive counselling about tinnitus and be told:

- tinnitus is common in those with a hearing impairment;
- it is not a disease, nor a symptom of a brain tumour etc.;
- with time most people adapt and live with their tinnitus.;
- it is very unlikely to get worse and is not an indicator of progressive hearing loss.

Background masking

Background masking suggestions are needed as part of strategies to lessen the awareness of tinnitus when it is troublesome. This is often when the patient is not wearing their hearing aid such as in the evening or in bed. At these times there is often little to distract their mind away from the tinnitus and the advantage of masking sounds may already have been discovered, such as having the TV/radio/stereo on. A small, cheap transistor radio or speaker set between stations or music under the pillow can be useful as it does not disturb the sleeping partner.

Tinnitus dominant symptom; first specialist consultation

If such a patient has an associated hearing impairment this will be managed with a hearing aid but usually with the object of lessening the awareness of tinnitus rather than improving the hearing. Occasionally some patients do not recognize that their hearing is impaired, particularly if only the higher frequencies are affected. This should be pointed out to them because it gives them an identifiable reason for their tinnitus. Management with a high-frequency emphasis hearing aid with an open mould should provide beneficial masking in such patients.

Patients without an obvious hearing impairment on pure tone audiometry (including the intermediate frequencies) should be told that despite this their tinnitus is likely to be caused by some minor malfunction of the hair cells in the cochlea which is not bad enough to be evident as a hearing impairment. This gives them a rational reason for having the tinnitus which in itself should not cause concern.

Both those with and without a hearing impairment in this group require some time spent on positive counselling. This is obviously best given by someone with an aura of experience (i.e. not a junior trainee) and the ability to inspire confidence. Provided time is available this should probably be done at the first visit. Specific enquiry ought to be made of the patient about their concerns so that these can be answered in addition to making the points listed above.

Whether an audiometric assessment is made of the tinnitus depends on whether the results can be used to reassure the patient. What has to be avoided is the use of investigations which might indicate uncertainty or concern on behalf of the clinician.

Background masking strategies are discussed and the patient reviewed several weeks later. At this stage, the majority are considerably less concerned by their tinnitus. Positive counselling is repeated with enquiry about any specific concerns the patient may still have at this stage. In those who are still having problems, a tinnitus masker to increase background noise should be considered and is often requested.

Tinnitus maskers

Tinnitus maskers are particularly of value in those that have normal hearing and are therefore unsuitable for a hearing aid. Maskers are also of value to those with a hearing aid at times when the aid is not being used such as in bed. Tinnitus maskers are of no real value to those with a profound or total impairment as they will not hear the masking sound.

Tinnitus maskers produce a continuous, broad-band noise whose frequency can be slightly but not greatly modified by adjusting a tone control, similar to that on a hearing aid (*Figure 14.1*). Like hearing aids, there are in-the-ear (ITE) and behind-the-ear (BTE) models, the former being more comfortable to wear in bed. The output can be varied. Models exist that can produce 90 dB SPL. The fact that the frequency spectrum of the masker is not that of the tinnitus is considered irrelevant.

In selecting a model, what the fitter does is: (a) ensure that the patient can hear the masker; (b) confirm that they find the masking a more acceptable noise than their tinnitus; and (c) ensure that by adjusting the volume control there is sufficient power to mask out the patient's tinnitus or at least make it less troublesome. Most patients use the masker below the total masking level.

Why then are tinnitus maskers acceptable, if all they do is substitute one noise for another? They would appear to act mainly as a psychological prop in that the masker is under the control of the user which is not the case with their own tinnitus. The placebo effect of having an instrument is considerable; the reported benefits in a recent cross-over study were as great with a placebo instrument as with a real tinnitus masker (Erlandsson *et al.*, 1987).

What proportion of patients are helped by tinnitus maskers is a difficult question to answer, because the characteristics of the patients who have been fitted with a masker are seldom reported and are unlikely to be representative of the average tinnitus sufferer because of the different referral patterns to specialized clinics which report their results. Probably in the region of 50 per cent get 'partial or total' relief from their symptoms (McFadden, 1982) but this requires a considerable amount of time being spent on counselling and on instructing the patient in the use of the masker. How much benefit such patients would get if a similar amount of time and effort was spent on counselling alone is unknown.

One of the simpler mistakes that can be made when providing a masker is to use an incorrect ear mould. The object is to mask the tinnitus but not to exclude outside sounds, so an open rather than a closed mould is preferred with BTE models.

Combination hearing aids and maskers are available that can be switched to either mode. Patients in general prefer two separate instruments which they swap as required.

Tinnitus dominant symptom; previous specialist consultation

This numerically small group of patients requires a considerable amount of consultation

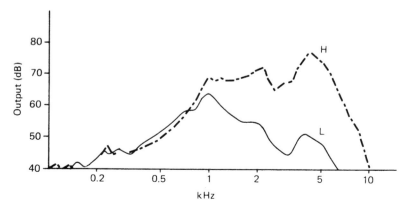

Figure 14.1 Typical maximum output of a tinnitus masker/sound generator. H = high tone setting; L = low tone setting

time. They tend to have introspective or obsessive personalities and sometimes have overt signs of depression. Having excluded the need for a psychiatric consultation the main objective is to try to change the patient's attitude and reaction to their tinnitus. This comes under the heading of tinnitus retraining therapy.

Tinnitus retraining therapy (TRT)

As the vast majority of patients with tinnitus are not particularly bothered by it, the reason that a few are must be because of their emotional reactions to it, there being no difference in the loudness or frequency spectrum of tinnitus in the two groups. Such patients have a vicious circle of negative responses (Jastreboff and Hazell, 1993) which needs to be broken. How this is best done is problematical but psychological counselling, biofeedback, relaxation therapy, hypnosis and more recently the use of maskers as 'retraining instruments' have been advocated. In these circumstances they are not called maskers but sound generators even though they are the same thing. All such techniques take place over a protracted period of time, often up to 2 years, by which time 70–80 per cent report the tinnitus to be less troublesome. There are no controlled studies to separate out specific advantages of such techniques, but what is common to all is someone with an interest in tinnitus and the time to spend with each patient.

Sound therapy

The principle here is that by repeated exposure to low level noise the auditory system adapts and finds intrusive noise less troublesome. This is achieved by wearing a sound generator (tinnitus masker) at an output where the patient hears both the masking sound and their tinnitus but is not intrusive enough to interfere with hearing. Hence a BTE sound generator with an open mould is used, usually binaurally. This therapy is continued daily for at least 8 hours for several months (up to 12) and many find that at the end of this 'retraining period' their tinnitus is less troublesome. Such retraining is one of the few options for those with hyperacusis, that is greater sensitivity to noise (see below).

Why sound therapy should work is unclear because everyday background noise must do the same thing. However, it has a high success rate such that in 70 per cent of cases the tinnitus is less intrusive and in a further 20 per cent there is virtual abolition of the tinnitus over a 2-year period. What is required is a controlled trial against counselling without sound therapy.

Hyperacusis management

Some individuals with tinnitus also have an increased sensitivity to sounds (hyperacusis) and so, for example, they say that they cannot go to work or out socially because they cannot stand the noise. Such symptoms are part of a spectrum of phonophobia which we all have to some extent. This is an irrational emotional dislike of certain sounds which, although quiet in terms of sound pressure levels, are intrusive, such as the TV on next door or the beat from a personal stereo.

Some patients with hyperacusis also have recruitment (see p. 2) but recruitment in a non-aided ear is seldom by itself a cause for hyperacusis. It is considered a higher cortical emotional response to sound. Counselling with the objective of retraining this emotional response to sound is necessary. Sound desensitization with sound generators (tinnitus maskers) is also thought to be of help. If the patient has a hearing aid, the maximal output ought to be adjusted to ensure that it is below the loudness discomfort level. In some patients automatic gain control by compression can be helpful. Whilst the wearing of ear plugs in some circumstances can be of value, their regular use ought to be discouraged as this will mitigate against the retraining of the central auditory system's handling of noise.

Non-proven therapies

Drug therapy

Unfortunately, to date no antitinnitus drug has been proven to be effective in randomized controlled trials, even though hope was raised of finding an oral analogue of lignocaine which can be beneficial when given intravenously (Martin and Colman, 1980). Night sedation can be given on a short term basis to overcome a crisis and obviously patients with psychiatric conditions merit medication on that account.

Surgery

It would seem reasonable to hope that surgery for a conductive hearing impairment might also alleviate any associated tinnitus by introducing previously unheard environmental sounds which would mask out the tinnitus or at least make it less noticeable. Reports on what happens to tinnitus after surgery are relatively few but it would appear that about 40 per cent of those who have successful surgery for otosclerosis will also be relieved of their tinnitus (Glasgold and Altman, 1965). If surgery is unsuccessful, there is a likelihood that the tinnitus will become more severe. So, if the primary aim is to relieve the tinnitus, it would be sensible in the first instance to provide a hearing aid rather than to operate on patients with a conductive hearing impairment.

It might be thought that for patients who are being 'driven to suicide', dividing the cochlear nerve might be an effective last resort. Not many centres perform this kind of surgery but there are now several reports on what has happened to the tinnitus of individuals who have had surgery for an acoustic neuroma (House and Brackman, 1981). In 50 per cent the tinnitus was 'worse', in 40 per cent 'better' and in 10 per cent 'the same'. Division of the cochlear nerve cannot therefore be recommended.

Most surgeons at the present time would not suggest inserting a cochlear implant primarily to relieve tinnitus but in 40 patients who were implanted by the House group for a hearing impairment, the severity of any associated tinnitus was reduced in 52 per cent, abolished in 27 per cent and made no worse in the remaining 21 per cent (House and Brackman, 1981).

■ Conclusions

- At least 15 per cent of adults have tinnitus at some time or other.
- By far the majority of these individuals will have an associated hearing impairment, no one aetiology for this being associated with a higher incidence of tinnitus.
- At present audiological assessment of tinnitus adds little to diagnosis or management.
- Positive counselling is required to tell the patient that tinnitus is common in those with a hearing impairment, that it is not a sign of progressive deafness or brain disease, and that though it might be troublesome the vast majority of individuals adapt and live with their tinnitus.
- Thankfully, only a small minority of patients are troubled by their tinnitus and in some there are associated personality problems.
- In those with troublesome tinnitus, a psychological appraisal may be useful in identifying individuals with psychiatric conditions.
- Tinnitus retraining therapy is the name given to a variety of techniques whose aim is to repeatedly counsel the patient and retrain their psychological reaction to the tinnitus.
- Tinnitus maskers are sometimes used in tinnitus retraining therapy as sound desensitizers, where their role is not to mask out the tinnitus but to retrain the brain.
- The currently available tinnitus maskers are most likely to give benefit because they are a psychological 'prop', rather than because they mask out the tinnitus.
- Medication may be useful for night sedation and for treating depression.
- Apart from this there is no specific tinnitus medication which can be taken orally that is of proven efficacy.

Further reading

Coles, R.R.A. (1997). Tinnitus. In *Adult Audiology*, Vol. 2, Chap. 18, Scott-Brown's Otolaryngology, 6th Edition. Butterworth-Heinemann, Oxford.

Vesterager, V. (1997). Tinnitus – investigation and management. *British Medical Journal*, **314**, 728–732.

15 Disequilibrium*

Introduction

Most otologists dread having to see a patient whose referral letter states that he has disequilibrium. There are many reasons why this is the case but it is mainly because they are uncertain as to what the potential diagnoses are and how to arrive at them. There is also an underlying fear that some life-threatening condition will be missed but this is extremely unlikely and, as a consequence, the majority of patients can be managed by reassurance and without the need for sophisticated investigations.

The prevalence of disequilibrium within the general population has never been accurately defined and the incidence in an ORL clinic will vary from hospital to hospital because of referral patterns. The syndrome or diagnosis ascribed depends primarily on how the clinician interprets the patient's symptoms and signs, as in the majority a definite pathology will never be demonstrated by objective means such as biopsy or radiology. For understandable reasons otologists will more frequently diagnose otological conditions than would a neurologist and vice versa. In a large series of 1000 individuals with dizziness seen by otologists and neurologists together, 45 per cent were postulated to have a neurological or vascular disorder, 25 per cent to have a purely peripheral disorder and in the remaining 30 per cent the site or type of disorder was indeterminate (Montandon and Hausler, 1984).

Many otologists see their role as deciding whether or not the disequilibrium is otological in origin but the main difficulty with this attitude is that disequilibrium cannot easily be broken down into otological and other causes. As will be discussed below, there are only a few conditions which can unequivocally be attributed to a particular site.

*Warning: This chapter should be taken in small doses by examination candidates as it may be dangerous to repeat.

Background physiology

Equilibrium is maintained by the cerebellum and central vestibular systems co-ordinating the sensory inputs from the vestibular system, the eyes and the proprioceptors in the muscles of the limbs, trunk and neck (*Figure 15.1*). Conventionally the vestibular system is divided into two parts, based on anatomy rather than on function. The peripheral vestibular system consists of the three semicircular canals, the macule, the saccule, the utrile and the vestibular divisions of the eighth cranial nerve. The central vestibular system consists of the neurological connections within the brain stem, cerebellum and cerebrum which process the sensory inputs from the peripheral vestibular, visual and proprioceptive systems.

The vascular supply of both the central and peripheral vestibular system is from the vertebro-basilar artery, so that if for any reason it is poorly perfused the brain stem, cerebellum and the peripheral system are all likely to be affected.

One of the advantages of space flights has been the ability to test some of the hypotheses as to how the components interact. Perhaps somewhat disappointingly, many of the concepts about the functions of the various parts of the peripheral vestibular system have not

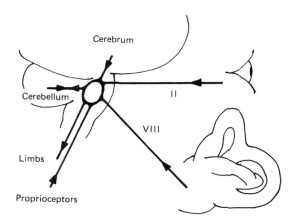

Figure 15.1 The sensory system responsible for maintaining balance

been confirmed (*Lancet* Editorial, 1984). Some fundamental rethinking is necessary but for diagnostic purposes it is important to remember that the distinction between the peripheral and the central vestibular system is an anatomical one. Functionally, it is one system with considerable interaction between the parts, effected by a complex afferent and efferent nervous system.

Background pathology

Disease can affect any part of parts of the system illustrated in *Figure 15.1* but for practical purposes disorders of the visual system are so rare that they can be discounted with the exception of congenital nystagmus. This should not be difficult to exclude because the patient will be aware that he has had eye problems since birth.

It is generally considered that the most likely part of the system to be affected will be the vestibular system in either its peripheral *or* central parts. This is incorrect for several reasons. Degenerative disorders of the proprioceptive system are fairly common and when

the vestibular system is affected *both* the central and the peripheral parts are likely to be involved. As the latter point may not be generally realized it is worthy of further comment.

Vascular causes are likely to be one of the more frequent causes of disequilibrium and as the brain stem, cerebellum and peripheral vestibular system are supplied by the vertebrobasilar artery, it is extremely likely that both parts will be affected by conditions which result in ischaemia. Thus, for example, hypotension (postural or drug induced), arteriosclerotic narrowing of the vertebro-basilar artery and osteoarthritic compression of the vertebral artery are as likely to affect several parts of the vestibular system as they are to affect one part alone.

Finally, though the site that is affected in a specific patient may be suspected it will not be possible in the majority of instances to prove this or to identify what is the underlying pathology. This inability to diagnose neurological pathology is not limited to individuals with disequilibrium and as a consequence the majority of patients will be ascribed a symptom/syndrome label rather than diagnosed as having a disease.

Symptom/syndrome labels

Endolymphatic hydrops

Endolymphatic hydrops is a well-documented entity occurring in about 5 per cent of human temporal bones with ear pathology. The main finding is bowing of Reissner's membrane into the scala vestibuli which is said, but never proven, to imply a continued increase in endolymphatic pressure. There is usually also distension of the membranes of the saccule and the macule but distension of the vestibular aqueduct or the endolymphatic sac has not been reported. In man the term sac is probably a misnomer as in 75 per cent of temporal bones the sac is a sinusoidal (*Figure 15.2*) rather than a bag-like structure (Plantenga and Browning, 1979).

In many instances there is no obvious reason why the hydrops has developed but in a considerable proportion of temporal bones, chronic otitis media, congenital syphilis and developmental abnormalities are also present. The hydrops is then considered to be a secondary phenomenon. In animals, hydrops has also been reported to occur following noise exposure and surgical obliteration of the vestibular aqueduct. It is interesting that such animals have not been reported to develop fluctuating hearing or vestibular problems. It is also interesting that in two-thirds of patients from whom bones with hydrops were taken, fluctuating hearing along with vestibular symptoms had *not* been noted during life (Plantenga, 1983).

It has been suggested that breaks in the continuity of Reissner's membrane are the pathological correlate of an episode of disequilibrium and fluctuating hearing. However,

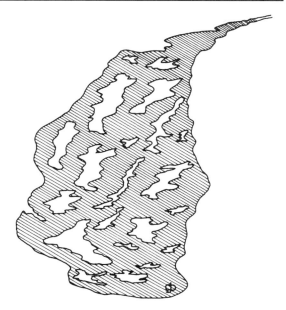

Figure 15.2 Human endolymphatic sac

such breaks could be preparation artefacts, especially as they are frequently detected and none of the individuals whose temporal bone had a ruptured Reissner's membrane is known to have died during an acute episode of disequilibrium.

At present endolymphatic hydrops cannot be diagnosed during life. Though narrowing and shortening of the vestibular aqueduct does occur in 70 per cent of bones with secondary hydrops, there is no evidence that bones with idiopathic hydrops are any different in this respect from normal.

Cupulolithiasis/canalothiasis

Schuknecht (1969) first described the histological occurrence of deposits, presumably displaced debris from the otoconia of the utricle, on the ampullae of the posterior semicircular canal. This he named cupulolithiasis and postulated that it was the histological correlate of benign paroxysmal positioning vertigo. In this condition patients report transient vertigo on moving the head into certain positions such as when lying down and rolling to the affected side. The clinical diagnosis is usually confirmed by a positive Hallpike test (see p. 206) accompanied by transient, fatiguable nystagmus. Nowadays a more commonly held view is that the debris is mobile and not attached to the ampulla of the posterior semicircular canal. The alternative name given is canalothiasis and, if the latter situation is indeed the case, repositioning manoeuvres (see p. 171) are a valid means of moving the debris back, hopefully permanently, to the utricle.

Clinical assessment of disequilibrium

In a patient with disequilibrium the clinician's first objective is to elucidate the patient's symptoms and decide which symptom complex/syndrome they best fit into. The second objective is to try to identify the responsible aetiology by asking some more general questions and by examining the patient. The limiting factor in achieving these two objectives is often the lack of time in a busy clinic. In these circumstances the natural reaction is to investigate the patient in the hope that this will provide the answer. In most instances such investigations will not and certainly not if considered on their own. A much better reaction would be to bring the patient back when time is available and complete the clinical assessment. If this were to be done most patients could be dealt with within 15 minutes and a few might take as long as 30 minutes, but in the majority there will be no need for investigations.

The following is a guideline for the average otologist in an ORL clinic rather than for a neuro-otologist in a specialist clinic. In many instances there will be little need to complete the entire protocol. So, for example, if a patient has had a previous stapedectomy, a 5 minute history and clinical examination is probably all that will be required.

What symptom complex/syndrome does the patient have?

The taking of a careful history is perhaps the single most important thing that the otologist does in a patient with disequilibrium. It is important for the otologist to elucidate the patient's symptoms himself and not to rely on a previous diagnosis made either by a doctor or the patient. At the end of the interview the otologist should be able to decide which symptom complex/syndrome (*Table 15.1*) the patient has.

The symptom complexes listed are neither comprehensive nor mutually exclusive but cover the majority of patients an otologist will see. Over the years some of these complexes have been ascribed names and this habit has led some to consider that syndromes such as vestibular neuronitis, positional vertigo and Ménière's syndrome are specific diseases caused by a certain pathology. This is not the case. Each is a syndrome for which there are many postulated and often conflicting theories regarding their aetiology and it is only occasionally that an individual with a syndrome will be found to have a definite disease. So, for example, in the majority of individuals acute labyrinthitis is idiopathic but in the occasional patient a herpetic rash will develop on the pinna. In the latter instance it is reasonable to suggest a viral aetiology, but it is wrong to suggest that all cases of acute labrynthitis are caused by viruses.

Peripheral vestibular symptoms/syndromes

At this stage it is worth describing a typical episode of peripheral vertigo and, as many otologists will have had experience of individuals with disequilibrium as a complication of ear surgery, this is a suitable model.

The patient will most often but not invariably complain of true vertigo, which is the sensation of rotation of the environment or of the patient rotating within the environment. The situation is usually made worse by head movement or shutting the eyes, which means that visual suppression of the symptoms is no longer possible. Initially there will be gross horizontal nystagmus, with the slow drift of the eyes

Table 15.1 Commoner symptom complexes/syndromes

Symptom complex	Syndrome
Peripheral vestibular:	
Acute vertigo alone	Vestibular neuronitis
Acute vertigo with hearing loss	Acute labyrinthitis
Episodic vertigo with or without hearing impairment	Chronic labyrinthitis
Episodic vertigo with or without hearing	Ménière's syndrome
Combined vestibular:	
Recurrent disequilibrium with positioning factors	Benign paroxysmal positioning vertigo (BPPV)
Recurrent disequilibrium on walking	
Recurrent disequilibrium with neurological symptoms (diplopia, disarthria, headache, etc.)	
Drop attacks/falls	
Proprioceptive:	
Inco-ordination on walking	
Neck movement initiated symptoms	
Psychological:	
Hysterical	
Atypical symptoms	

going to the side of the affected ear and with the fast recovery beat going to the other side.

The patient's symptoms and nystagmus usually subside over a few days due to central compensation. During this phase the nystagmus may be provoked by sudden head movement but this is almost invariably accompanied by vertigo. The symptoms settle with time though there may be further acute, milder, episodes. Following stapedectomy these symptoms are usually considered to be due to perilymph leaks. Once the symptoms have subsided a residual balance disorder can often be detected by the patient being unstable when walking heel to toe with the eyes shut.

Individuals with a peripheral disorder due to other aetiologies usually have many features in common with the above typical history. The additional presence of a unilateral hearing loss, tinnitus or the sensation of fullness in the ear makes a peripheral cause more likely but by no means certain because of the high prevalence of these symptoms in individuals who do not have disequilibrium. If there is a close relationship between the onset of the disequilibrium and the other otological symptoms then the likelihood of a peripheral aetiology is, of course, increased.

Having decided that the patient's symptoms fall into the pattern of a pure peripheral disorder it is a matter of definition what syndrome, if any, is ascribed.

Vestibular neuronitis is usually taken to be an acute episode of peripheral type disequilibrium but without any other otological or neurological symptoms. Most would consider that such an episode has been caused by a viral or vascular condition and a large proportion of the patients will never have any further trouble but some may proceed to develop vertebro-basilar ischaemia, chronic labyrinthitis or multiple sclerosis.

Acute labyrinthitis is similar to vestibular neuronitis but, in addition, there may or may not be other otological symptoms such as tinnitus and hearing impairment. Whether there is any real pathological difference between vestibular neuronitis and acute labyrinthitis is doubtful.

Chronic labyrinthitis is essentially recurrent episodes of vertigo with or without other permanent otological symptoms.

Ménière's syndrome is the symptom complex of episodes of vertigo, lasting minutes to hours, and often associated with a sensation of fullness in one ear and an increase in the loudness of the tinnitus in that ear. Whilst a deterioration in the hearing during an episode is required to satisfy the classical description of Ménière's (Alford, 1972) this is not always present. What is usually present is a sensorineural hearing impairment, which classically is greater at the lower frequencies (*Figure 15.3*) rather than at the higher frequencies. The natural history of the condition is that the

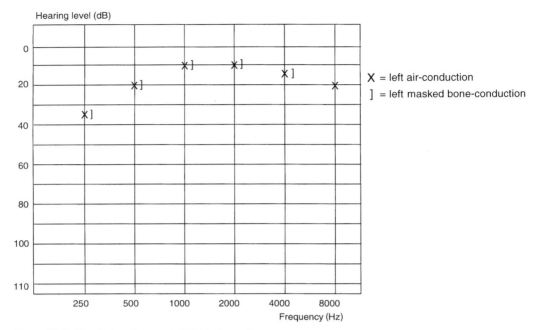

Figure 15.3 Classical audiogram in Ménière's syndrome

episodes of vertigo decrease in frequency with time and disappear. In a few patients this unfortunately does not occur and the sensori-neural hearing impairment increases in degree.

The pathological correlate of Ménière's syndrome is considered to be endolymphatic hydrops (see p. 157). Unfortunately, it is not possible to diagnose endolymphatic hydrops during life, it remaining a condition which can only be confirmed by histological sectioning of the temporal bone. Contrary to earlier reports (Stahle and Wilbrand, 1974) radiology, including tomography, does not distinguish patients with Ménière's disease from normal individuals (Kraus and Dubois, 1979). Glycerol dehydration tests have been advocated as a reliable way of detecting hydrops, the theory being that dehydration causes a reduction in endolymphatic pressure which is reflected by an improvement in the pure tone thresholds. Many papers have reported improvement in the pure tone and speech thresholds but these are frequently within test/retest error and it is probable that these patients were led to believe that their hearing might improve. The psychological aspects have to be controlled for as it has been found that when the same

patients are told that their hearing will deteriorate after dehydration it will do so (Thomsen and Vesterhauge, 1979). In this study, in only two of the 15 patients with Ménière's syndrome did the hearing improve when the individuals were told that their hearing was expected to deteriorate. Even if a patient's hearing does improve, there is no evidence that this is because of hydrops: there are many other possible biochemical explanations.

It has been suggested that Ménière's disease is the clinical correlate of endolymphatic hydrops which presents as episodes of fluctuating hearing and vertigo (i.e. Ménière's syndrome). Unfortunately this chain of thought has several defects in it. In etymological terms a disease is defined as an abnormality of the body or its function which may or may not be associated with symptoms and signs. Thus, a cerebral tumour is a disease which may on occasions be associated with epilepsy (a symptom). This does not mean that all individuals with epilepsy have a cerebral tumour; the vast majority do not.

There is indeed evidence that some individuals who, during life, had symptoms in keeping with Ménière's syndrome histologically had endolymphatic hydrops in their temporal bones. In these particular individuals it is therefore valid to consider that they had a disease process and to call it Ménière's disease but it would be wrong to state as a result of this finding that all individuals with Ménière's syndrome will have endolymphatic hydrops and therefore Ménière's disease. The reasons why this would be invalid are as follows. The proportion of individuals with Ménière's syndrome who have endolymphatic hydrops has never been reported, primarily because there is no proven way of diagnosing hydrops during life. Several ways have been suggested as to how hydrops might be diagnosed but no study has reported whether there is a correlation between the results of such investigations and histological hydrops. It is well recognized that not all individuals who, post-mortem, are found to have hydrops had episodic vertigo during life and indeed it is only about one-third of such individuals who had symptoms in keeping with Ménière's syndrome.

The chain of evidence is as invalid as it would be to state the following. Coronary artery stenosis is a pathology found post-mortem in some individuals who, during life, had symptoms of chest pain, so it follows that all individuals with chest pain will have coronary artery stenosis. This sequence of statements is patently untrue and what makes this situation easy to resolve is that there are reliable ante-mortem means of diagnosing coronary artery stenosis. So, though some individuals with fluctuating hearing and episodic vertigo may have hydrops, it is as yet unknown what the proportion is and as it is impossible to diagnose hydrops during life it is correspondingly impossible to diagnose Ménière's disease during life. The situation would be most easily resolved by reporting the pathological findings in individuals with idiopathic vestibular symptoms and fluctuating hearing.

It could be argued that it does not really matter if the term Ménière's disease is used. This is not the case. The misuse has given rise to a series of misdirected operations for endolymphatic hydrops in the belief that all individuals with Ménière's syndrome will have Ménière's disease, that is endolymphatic hydrops. Now it may well be that a proportion of individuals with Ménière's syndrome will have hydrops but it will not be all of them. The continued use of the term Ménière's disease only strengthens the unfounded opinion that individuals with Ménière's syndrome will invariably have hydrops.

Central vestibular symptoms/syndromes

Pathology which solely affects the central vestibular system is relatively uncommon, tumours and infarcts of the brain stem or cerebellum being the main conditions. Such conditions are unlikely to cause only imbalance. Other conditions such as ischaemia are as likely to affect both the central and peripheral parts as they are the central part alone. The following aspects in the history would suggest that there was a central component to the symptom-complex:

- If there is disordered balance or difficulty in locomotion.
- If there are neurological symptoms such as black-outs, falls, limb weakness, migraine, blurring of vision or slurring of speech.
- If the imbalance continues over several weeks or months, in contradistinction to peripheral disorders which typically last hours or days. This is because central compensation occurs in peripheral disorders but not in central conditions.

Combined peripheral and central vestibular symptoms/syndromes

Perhaps the most common symptom which would suggest a combined peripheral and central aetiology is when a change in head position provokes the disequilibrium.

Many consider that disequilibrium occasioned by a change in head position implies an otological (i.e. peripheral) pathology. This is by no means the case as it can be caused by factors other than an inappropriate input from the peripheral vestibular system. Thus, conditions which result in ischaemia of both the central and peripheral vestibular system are often made worse by a change in head position. Postural hypotension, vertebro-basilar arteriosclerosis or compression from an osteoarthritis cervical spine are common examples and subclavian artery steal syndrome is an uncommon example. If the patient has more than vestibular symptoms, such as diplopia, dysarthria, limb weakness or loses consciousness, the area involved due to the ischaemia is obviously more extensive.

Another common aetiology that has to be considered for positioning problems is inappropriate input from the sensory organs, either the proprioceptors or the vestibular labyrinth (see below). Finally, it is not uncommon for disequilibrium which is a result of cerebellar, brain stem and cerebello-pontine angle tumours to be provoked by positioning factors.

It can thus be seen that it is important to enquire if the symptoms come on when the neck is extended (to look up) or twisted (to look round) or when there is a change in body position without neck movement such as getting up from a bed or from a chair.

Proprioceptive system symptoms/syndromes

A frequent problem that can be attributable to a faulty proprioceptor system is the lack or co-ordination that often accompanies ageing. Most elderly individuals have poorer 'righting' reflexes than they used to have so that simple incidents, like tripping over the edge of a pavement, result in a fall. These falls are *not* a result of a vestibular disorder or of a transient ischaemic attack though the fall may result in a head injury with unconsciousness.

Another frequent and increasingly recognized problem attributable to the proprioceptive system is disequilibrium which is occasioned by head movements causing an inappropriate input from the proprioceptors in the neck. The differential diagnosis of position-induced disequilibrium is complicated but it is important to repeat that otological (peripheral) vestibular upsets are by no means the only cause of such problems.

In comparison to the above age-related degenerative, proprioceptive disorders, distinct pathologies such as tabes dorsalis do not usually present as disequilibrium but rather as locomotion problems. As such they should be comparatively easy to identify.

Psychological symptoms/syndromes

Psychological causes of disequilibrium should not be forgotten and indeed in some practices overbreathing is reported to be the commonest cause of disequilibrium. The history of what actually happens, especially if confirmed by a relative or friend, should make the diagnosis obvious.

Another common complaint is the feeling of imbalance when up high, such as climbing on to a chair. This again should be easily identified from the history. What is less easy to identify is a psychological background for atypical symptoms. If at any time the symptoms are rather vague or at variance with the otologist's experience of typical histories of disequilibrium, the possibility of a functional disorder should be considered. Obviously the more experience the otologist has the easier it is to suspect a non-organic cause and be confident of it.

Does the patient have an identifiable aetiology?

Having elucidated the patient's symptoms, an attempt is made to identify any definite or postulated aetiology by asking some general questions and carrying out a clinical examination. In most instances none will be identified. Before this is discussed it is perhaps worthwhile discussing the difference between a definite and a postulated aetiology.

Definite aetiology

Under this heading come conditions (*Table 15.2*) which are strongly suggested because of a direct cause/effect relationship (e.g. barotrauma, aminoglycosides), because of the results of examination (e.g. positive fistula test in chronic otitis media), because of the results of investigations (e.g. MRI showing infarcts and tumours) or because of operative findings

Table 15.2 Diseases that can cause disequilibrium

Peripheral:
  Chronic otitis media
  Ear surgery
  Barotrauma
  Temporal bone fracture
  Perilymph leak
  Aminoglycosides
Peripheral and central:
  Drugs
  Cerebello-pontine angle tumours
  Vertebro-basilar ischaemia
  Multiple sclerosis
  Whiplash injuries
Central:
  Brain stem and cerebellar tumours
  Brain stem and cerebellar infarcts

(e.g. cerebello-pontine angle tumour). The relationship between the patient's symptoms and the pathology is then hardly in doubt. Unfortunately, taking drugs and chronic otitis media are common, yet though they cause disequilibrium in some patients, in the majority they do not. Therefore the clinician should not assume that when present these factors are the cause of the symptoms and alternative reasons should also be considered.

Postulated aetiologies

Within this category (*Table 15.3*) are ear pathologies such as endolymphatic hydrops and cupulolithiasis which cannot be diagnosed during life. Both of these have been histologically described in temporal bones and have been correlated with the symptoms the patient is reported to have had during life. This does not mean that if a patient has these symptoms they must have the corresponding pathology. There are many other potential aetiologies for any symptom so, for example, it would seem reasonable in a patient with episodic vertigo and a fluctuating sensorineural hearing impairment to postulate that intermittent hypo-perfusion of the vertebro-basilar artery would be as likely to be the cause as endolymphatic hydrops. There are also many explanations other than cupulolithiasis for disequilibrium that is brought about by changes in head position. So until it becomes possible to reliably diagnose endolymphatic hydrops and cupulolithiasis these conditions can only be postulated.

In the second category of postulated aetiologies are general diseases that are diagnosable, but if an individual patient has such a disease its relationship with the disequilibrium can only be postulated. An example of this category is diabetes which is a definite disease, but if a patient has both disequilibrium and diabetes are the two related? It can be suggested that they are, but currently there is no way of proving it.

Table 15.3 Conditions postulated to be associated with disequilibrium

Ear disease:
   Endolymphatic hydrops
   Cupulolithiasis
General disease:
   Diabetes
   Hypertension
   Thyroid dysfunction
   Anaemia

General history

It is important to ask the patient certain questions relating to past events that may be connected to the development/onset of the disequilibrium. Specific areas of concern are outlined below.

Areas of concern

Previous ear disease or surgery

The questions to ask should be obvious to an otologist, the main aim being to exclude the likelihood of a fistula.

Recent aeroplane flight or diving

These should be enquired about and if related to the onset of the disequilibrium a round window fistula or decompression sickness is likely (see p. 68).

Previous head or neck injury

There is usually a definite time relationship between the onset of the disequilibrium and the trauma. The diagnostic difficulty is to distinguish between a temporal bone fracture and a whiplash injury to the brain stem. Whiplash injuries of the brain stem due to sudden uncontrolled movement of the cervical spine would appear to be relatively easy to sustain, especially in road traffic accidents. A temporal bone fracture is only likely if there has been a definite temporo-parietal injury (see p. 67).

General disease

The majority of individuals will know whether they have any of the generalized disorders listed in *Table 15.3*. The fact that a patient has one of these diseases does not mean that it is the cause of the symptoms, it only makes it a postulated factor.

Current medication

Nearly 300 drugs have been reported by the manufacturers to be associated with dizziness or vertigo and this number is too many to memorize. Thankfully, in many instances the drugs are not responsible but the only way to prove this is to stop them or to change to a different pharmacological group of drugs.

Previous medication

The most important drugs to enquire about which the patient may have taken in the past are the aminoglycosides. It is rare nowadays in developed countries for vestibulotoxic aminoglycosides to be prescribed except in hospital practice in patients who are severely ill, are on renal dialysis or have been severely burned. The history in such patients is usually clear cut, there being a definite relationship between being given the aminoglycosides and developing vestibular symptoms.

Otological examination

Otoscopy

This should be directed towards excluding chronic otitis media and, if suggested by the history, a temporal bone fracture. In the acute stage of the latter there will be either blood or CSF in the external auditory canal or a haemotympanum. In the resolved stage, the external auditory canal may be narrowed or there may be an obvious step in the posterior canal wall at the site of the fracture.

Fistula test

If otological pathology is detected then a fistula test should be performed by increasing the pressure intermittently in the external auditory canal using finger pressure on the tragus. The test is considered positive if this induces vertigo along with a few beats of nystagmus. Such a finding does not imply that there is an actual fistula in the conventional understanding of a channel through which fluid can exit. It is more likely that the bone overlying the semicircular canals has been eroded and the membranous labyrinth exposed. A change in pressure will cause symptoms because the fluid in the membranous canal is displaced. Unfortunately, a negative test does not exclude a fistula because mechanical factors could have prevented the change in pressure being transmitted to it.

Hearing assessment

Clinical tests of hearing are aimed at identifying an asymmetrical sensorineural hearing impairment to exclude an acoustic neuroma. If such an impairment is suspected then a pure tone audiogram should be requested both to confirm this and to ensure that it is not caused by a conductive defect. If an otological condition is considered unlikely, there would seem little point in performing audiometry, though for many otologists this is a necessary ritual which has to be carried out.

Ocular examination

There are several different reasons why the eyes should be examined and it could be argued that more information will be gained from doing this than from doing anything else.

Ocular palsies

The eye movements should first be assessed to detect IIIrd, IVth and VIth cranial nerve palsies which would suggest intracranial pathology.

Nystagmus

Nystagmus, which is an involuntary oscillation of the eyes, should be looked for, there being several different patterns which can be identified. By far the commonest has a fast horizontal component followed by a slow drift of the eyes back to the starting position. By convention the direction of the nystagmus is described by the direction of the fast component. Nystagmus can be either physiological or pathological.

Physiological nystagmus

This will be present in 75 per cent of normal individuals if the iris in each eye deviates horizontally further than the punctum of the lacrimal sac. *Figure 15.4* shows the outer limits of permitted eye deviation to detect pathological nystagmus. The other common types of physiological nystagmus are those produced by optokinetic and caloric stimulation (see below).

The main types of pathological nystagmus are congenital, spontaneous, and positional or positioning provoked.

Congenital nystagmus

This is easily differentiated from spontaneous nystagmus because abnormal eye movements will have been present since childhood. Congenital nystagmus disappears when the patient's eyes are viewed through Frenzel glasses, which remove visual fixation.

Spontaneous nystagmus

This is distinguished from positional or positioning nystagmus in that it is present when the patient is sitting still and there has been no external stimulus. Spontaneous nystagmus is enhanced by the removal of eye fixation and can sometimes only be detected when Frenzel glasses are worn. Increasing degrees of severity of spontaneous nystagmus are recognized.

- *First degree:* Present only when the eyes are deviated in the direction of the fast component.
- *Second degree:* Present on central gaze.
- *Third degree:* Present when the eyes are deviated in the direction of the slow component.

It is possible to record many other aspects of spontaneous nystagmus in the hope of identifying the site of the primary pathology. The average otologist is likely to find this rather complicated, but if the following rules are applied they will be correct on most occasions.

- If the patient has spontaneous nystagmus during an episode of disequilibrium then it is almost certainly caused by a peripheral (otological) condition.
- In a patient with spontaneous nystagmus, the pathology is almost certainly central in origin if the patient does not have disequilibrium at the time.
- The commonest cause of spontaneous

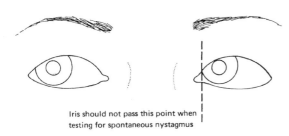

Iris should not pass this point when testing for spontaneous nystagmus

Figure 15.4 The limit of the punctum which the iris should not pass when testing for spontaneous nystagmus

nystagmus is current drug therapy. Barbiturates, benzodiazepines and phenytoin are the most likely culprits and they could well be being taken for the disequilibrium.

- Spontaneous nystagmus of peripheral origin usually fatigues.

Fundoscopy

The fundi should be examined for evidence of papilloedema, but the inexperienced should not be bold in interpreting the findings especially if mydriatics to dilate the iris have not been used. It could be that this is where spontaneous nystagmus is first detected because fundoscopy may remove visual fixation.

Positioning testing

The presence of positional or positioning nystagmus should be ascertained, the difference between the two being that the former is occasioned by the head being in a specific position whereas the latter is occasioned by the head being moved fairly rapidly to a specific position. This distinction is perhaps rather academic, it being more important to ascertain the role of neck movement. Positioning tests are described in Appendix IX.

If positional or positioning nystagmus is provoked, the next question is how to interpret the results. If neck extension is the main provoking factor then either vertebral artery compression from an osteoarthritic cervical spine or inappropriate proprioceptor input from the stretch receptors in the neck is likely. If head position or positioning is a factor then ischaemia of part of the entire vestibular system or specific peripheral disorders are possible. The presence of vertigo along with nystagmus is usually taken to indicate a peripheral disorder and is commonly labelled as benign paroxysmal positioning vertigo (BPPV). However, it must be remembered that one in three individuals with proven cerebellar disease will also get positioning vertigo (Harrison and Ozsahinoglu, 1972) and unfortunately making a distinction between the types of nystagmus provoked (e.g. central nystagmus is said to have no latency and to be non-fatiguable) is of minimal diagnostic value (Barber, 1975).

Neurological examination

A full neurological examination is not necessary in everyone and unless neurological symptoms are present, a screening examination will be performed. What this should include is uncertain but the following categories of examination should be considered.

Stance and gait

Many tests come into this category. The *Unterberger* test gets the patient to mark time by stepping on the spot with the eyes closed and the arms stretched out with the palms facing upwards. If the patient can do this without falling or turning there are essentially no balance problems.

In testing *head/toe gait* the patient is asked to walk with their eyes open, putting one foot, heel-to-toe, in front of the other. Most normal individuals can do this fairly well. Provided an individual is not in an acute episode of disequilibrium, a central component to the disorder is likely if they cannot perform this task.

Many would carry out a *Romberg* test which involves getting the patient to stand with their feet together and then to close their eyes. The test is positive if they are imbalanced. This test is only really relevant during an acute episode of disequilibrium when it will help elucidate the role of visual suppression.

Cerebellar function

Others would routinely perform a test of cerebellar function such as finger-nose pointing or rapidly pronating and supinating the hands.

Cranial nerves

The cochlear division of the VIIIth nerve will already have been assessed by testing the hearing as will the IIIrd, IVth and VIth cranial nerves by testing the ocular movement. The Vth (trigeminal) nerve is conventionally assessed by testing for corneal reflexes. However, the results of this are unreliable for many reasons but mainly because of the gross variability in the stimulus. It is better to ask if the patient has noticed any change in sensation on one side of the face. The VIIth (facial) nerve is tested by getting the patient to wrinkle the brow, shut the eyes, smile and whistle. The IXth (glossopharyngeal) nerve is tested by prodding the back of the throat on either side to elicit a gag reflex. The Xth (vagal) nerve is assessed by enquiring about voice disorders, and listening to the voice, and looking at movements of the soft palate for asymmetrical displacement. The XIth (accessory) nerve is tested by getting the patient to raise their shoulders with the examiner putting pressure on them or by assessing sternomastoid muscle contraction against head pressure. The XIIth (hypoglossal) nerve is tested by observing tongue movements. In a baby the tongue deviates to the contralateral side.

Cardiovascular examination

Which aspects of the cardiovascular system need to be examined will depend on whether there are any suggestive symptoms. In everyone, hypertension and cardiac arrhythmias should be excluded but it is doubtful if routine auscultation of the neck is of value.

Further investigations

None

At this stage the majority of patients require no further investigations. This is because most of the definite or postulated aetiologies will have been identified or excluded by taking a history and examining the patient.

The following is a list of the definite pathologies, taken from *Table 15.2*, whose diagnosis might be aided by further investigations. The list is short and the majority are diagnosed by radiology. None is diagnosed by caloric testing.

- Brain stem tumours
- Cerebellar tumours
- Cerebello-pontine tumours
- Brain stem and cerebellar infarction
- Vertebro-basilar ischaemia

If none of these is suspected there would appear little point in carrying out any investigations.

Radiology

The type of patients who are likely to require radiological investigations are those with the following:

- Neurological signs and increased intracranial pressure in order to exclude a space-occupying lesion. This will most likely be by MRI scanning because of its ability to assess soft tissue.
- Vertigo which is associated with a unilateral sensorineural hearing loss in order to exclude a cerebello-pontine angle tumour. Whether this is done by CT with contrast or MRI depends mainly on availability (see p. 61).
- Disequilibrium potentially due to vertebro-basilar artery compression. If neck extension produces disequilibrium radiological investigations are only warranted on the rare occasions that surgery is being contemplated. Under these circumstances arteriography is the investigation of choice.

Biochemistry/haematology/serology

Individuals with previously undiagnosed general disease will usually have symptoms in addition to their disequilibrium. Investigation is obviously then mandatory but it is doubtful whether routine biochemistry, haematology or serology is necessary.

Caloric testing

Traditionally the main reason for performing caloric tests is to confirm whether there is a peripheral component to the disequilibrium. This is not too difficult to ascertain from the history and the main defect of these tests is that when the symptoms are of presumed peripheral origin such as in Ménière's syndrome the tests are frequently normal. The tests will certainly indicate whether there is an unequal response from the two peripheral vestibular systems and suggest which side is affected. In coming to any conclusions the incidence of unequal responses in the population who do not have peripheral disorders has to be taken into account.

Caloric tests will never help identify which disease process is responsible within the peripheral or central vestibular system, nor do the results affect the management.

Ice-cold caloric testing

If all that is required to be known is whether caloric stimulation produces symptoms similar to those a patient is experiencing and whether there is relative hypofunction of one peripheral labyrinthine system compared to the other, it is not necessary to perform hot and cold calorics. Ice-cold calorics can be relatively easily performed in the clinic by the otologist, the only disadvantage being that they are slightly more unpleasant for the patient because iced water is used. If any more information is required, and it is argued that in a non-specialist clinic it is not, then a full vestibular test battery can be performed. The method of performing a hot and cold caloric test is essentially similar except for the temperature of the water.

The patient is seated on a couch with the head 30 degrees from the horizontal and 2 ml of ice-cold water are slowly instilled into the ear canal via a syringe and kept there for 20 seconds. The water is then drained out into a receptacle and the eyes observed for nystagmus in the straight ahead position. The duration of any nystagmus is timed with a stopwatch from the moment the water was instilled. The relative strength of the nystagmus is noted. If vertigo is provoked, the patient is asked if this is similar to his own symptoms though the caloric stimulus is likely to be more severe. The other ear is tested after waiting 5 minutes.

The following conclusions can be drawn, provided the cold water has been correctly instilled and this can be ascertained by asking the patient if they temporarily became dull of hearing due to water loading of the tympanic membrane. The disequilibrium is likely to be otological in origin if:

- the symptoms that are provoked are similar to the patient's symptoms;
- there is a difference in the duration of the nystagmus between the ears of greater than 30 seconds; and
- the affected ear is the one with the shorter response and often the lesser degree of nystagmus.

Electronystagmography

The additional use of electronystagmography in caloric testing allows nystagmus to be recorded both with the eyes open and closed and the eye movements to be measured, but it adds little to the diagnostic capacity of the test.

So, outside a neuro-otological clinic, calorics and electronystagmography have a minimum role. Even in a neuro-otological clinic they are more often a toy than an aid to diagnosis or management.

Glycerol dehydration

Frequently performed in the past with the object of diagnosing endolymphatic hydrops, its validity has never been proven and because of the considerable influence of suggestion in the results it is not frequently performed nowadays.

Electrocochleography

The theory is that the ratio of the summating and action potentials (SP/AP) ratio is increased and the coupler is broadened in endolymphatic hydrops. Though some strongly advocate the use of electrocochleography, most would generally feel that the test lacks sensitivity and specificity, and thus adds little to making the diagnosis or affecting decisions about management.

Management

By far the majority of individuals will be managed in a non-specific manner because a definite pathology is seldom identified. Even if an otological condition is diagnosed, non-specific measures are often instigated in the first instance in the hope that the symptoms will resolve spontaneously. The exception is if a definite central pathology such as a tumour is identified. The management in such cases is outside the scope of this text.

Non-specific management

Reassurance

Those who do *not* have neurological or cardiovascular disease can be confidently reassured that their symptoms will get less severe and most likely disappear with time. In the interim, any provoking factors such as sudden head movements should be avoided. The majority of patients will be relieved to be told that they do not have a brain tumour, that they have not had a stroke and that their blood pressure is normal. Non-specific vestibular exercises may be recommended but this is mainly for the psychological support they give rather than because they hasten resolution.

Unfortunately in those with definite neurological or cardiovascular disease such reassurance cannot be given as the symptoms are most often progressive.

Supportive medication

It is by no means necessary that a patient with disequilibrium be given supportive medication. This is for many reasons but mainly because medication is ineffective in a high proportion of patients and the side-effects can be worse than the condition being treated. The latter applies particularly to the elderly in whom, if the medication is discontinued, there can often be a marked improvement in the balance problems.

Some of the various drugs available for prescription are listed in *Table 15.4* and, contrary to what the advertisers may say, there is minimal evidence that one drug is superior to another nor is one more effective for a specific condition than another. All these drugs can be taken orally and those marked with an asterisk can also be given intramuscularly or as a suppository. Medication absorbed via the skin from patches is advocated by some but perhaps the best way for a patient to take medication if they are feeling sick and perhaps vomiting is by buccal absorption from a tablet placed between the upper lip and gum and left to dissolve (e.g. prochlorperazine or Buccastem).

Medication, if given at all, is most likely to be effective for episodes of disequilibrium that are likely to last for hours or days such as following middle ear surgery or acute labyrinthitis. In these circumstances a sedative side-effect can be an advantage. In patients whose episodes of disequilibrium lasts seconds or minutes, therapy for the acute episodes is pointless and the question is whether continuous prophylactic therapy reduces the frequency and severity of such episodes. The evidence that any of the drugs do this better than a placebo, in the majority of patients, is weak.

Exercise therapy

It is understandable that patients whose symptoms are aggravated by position or movement will try and avoid bringing on their symptoms by becoming immobile or inactive. There is a strong argument against encouraging this as the majority of vestibular symptoms resolve with time, presumably due in a large proportion of cases to central compensation. Avoidance of symptoms could then, in theory, delay this process.

Cawthorne and Cooksey developed exercises to hasten recovery from vestibular symptoms in the early days of otosclerosis surgery when this was common. These exercises or one of the many alternative regimens are now suggested for those with an acute episode due to any cause and to encourage movement in those with recurrent position provoked episodes (Cawthorne and Cooksey, 1997).

Specific management: Ménière's syndrome

In a condition in which the symptoms are episodic and self-resolving with time, great care has to be exercised in evaluating whether management is effective. When surgery is being studied the ideal would be to have a randomly allocated control group having a placebo operation. This would control for the not inconsiderable psychological effect of surgery which is demonstrated by the high success rate of operations, such as grommet insertion, where it is difficult to conceive how

Table 15.4 Non-specific medication for disequilibrium

Drug category	Drug name	Proprietary name
Antihistamines		
	Cinnerazine	Stugeron
	Cyclizine	Valoid
	Dimenhydrinate	Dramamine
	Mepyramine	Anthisan
	Promethazine	Phenergan
Phenothiazides		
	Chlorpromazine*	Largactil
	Prochlorperazine*	Stemetil/Vertigon/ Buccastem
	Thiethylperazine*	Torecan
Others		
	Betahistidine	Serc
	Scopolamine	

*Can also be given intramuscularly or as a suppository

such a procedure could benefit a vestibular disorder.

Various surgical procedures have been proposed which can be classified as to whether preservation of hearing is an aim, which it usually is, or whether the hearing is already so affected by the disease that its destruction is acceptable.

Hearing preservation operations include:

- Grommet insertion
- Cortical mastoidectomy
- Endolymphatic sac decompression
- Endolymphatic sac drainage
- Vestibular nerve section

Hearing destructive operations include:

- Labyrinthectomy
- Aminoglycoside perfusion of the middle ear

Hearing preservation operations

Vestibular nerve section is virtually 100 per cent effective in abolishing vertigo but requires a retrosigmoid or middle cranial fossa operation. The other operations in this category are difficult to understand on a physiological/pathological basis. Sac decompression is based on the premise that hydrops affects the sac, which it does not. Sac drainage operations are based on the premise that a drainage tube can be inserted into a bag-like sac. Histologically, because of its size and anatomical configuration (*Figure 15.2*), this is virtually impossible.

Hearing preservation surgery in general reports relief of symptoms in around 70 per cent of patients. Controlled studies are rare, but a randomized study has reported the effects of endolymphatic sac decompression against a placebo operation in the form of a superficial simple mastoidectomy (Thomsen *et al.*, 1981). After 6 months, 70 per cent of subjects in both groups reported relief of vertigo. No other controlled study of surgical management of otological vertigo has been identified, but most uncontrolled studies report a response rate in the region of 70 per cent. As such it must be regretfully concluded there is no proven surgical management for idiopathic peripheral vertigo which preserves the hearing.

The placebo effects of surgery should not be dismissed altogether, because it can be difficult to achieve similar placebo response rates by non-surgical means. What it means, however, is that as minor an operation as possible should be performed and a post-auricular incision would seem a reasonable procedure.

Hearing destructive procedures

Hearing destructive procedures should not be carried out unless after considerable thought. This is because in patients with troublesome Ménière's, the condition not infrequently affects both ears. Obviously if there is no residual hearing, a labyrinthectomy can be carried out either via the oval window or via the mastoid. Some would argue that aminoglycoside perfusion of the middle ear is unlikely to damage the hearing, provided the dosage is carefully controlled and a vestibular-toxic (gentamicin) rather than a cochleotoxic drug is used. Whilst this may be the case in some hands, hearing loss in up to 30 per cent of patients has been reported (Commins and Nedzeliki, 1996).

Specific management: Otological fistulae

A perilymph fistula following barotrauma, head injury or oval window surgery usually heals spontaneously. The management is at first conservative, but in the few whose symptoms continue after 7–10 days or in those who have had recurrent episodes, surgical sealing of the fistula is usually suggested, though it carries the not inconsiderable risk of cochlear damage.

Though not a true fistula, exposure of the membrane of the lateral semicircular canal by chronic otitis media is usually taken to indicate a high risk of intracranial infection. As such, surgical eradication of the disease is advocated but there is debate as to whether the diseased tissue should be removed from the area overlying the semicircular canal.

Specific management: Benign paroxysmal positioning vertigo

Canalothiasis or cupulolithiasis is the presumed pathological correlate in patients with the symptoms of benign paroxysmal positioning vertigo confirmed by a positive Hallpike test. Conceptually, if the otoliths are free, they could be dispersed from the posterior canal and perhaps even moved back to their presumed site of origin in the utricle.

Exercises that repeatedly provoke the symptoms (e.g. Cooksey–Cawthorne, Norre and Beckers, 1997) are reported to decrease symptoms either by dispersing the particles or by encouraging central compensation. The Epley and Semont manoeuvres on the other hand are more complex, going through a series of positions which theoretically move the particles round the posterior canal to the utricle. The reported results are impressive, with 80 per cent or more of cases being resolved after one manoeuvre (Beynon, 1997).

Singular nerve section via the middle ear is a surgical procedure with a 70 per cent response rate that some advocate. Overall it must be remembered that the majority of patients with this syndrome resolve spontaneously with time.

■ Conclusions

- It is conventional to consider disequilibrium to arise from the proprioceptive, vestibular or visual systems.
- Disorders of the proprioceptive system are fairly common and are likely to be the reason why older individuals often fall when they are momentarily put off balance. The history should identify this type of problem.
- In comparison, neurological conditions affecting the proprioceptive system are rare and should be identified by the associated locomotor symptoms and neurological signs.
- The peripheral vestibular system consists of the vestibular nerve, the semicircular canals, the macule and the saccule.
- The central vestibular system comprises the connections of the peripheral vestibular, the visual and the proprioceptive systems within the brain stem, cerebellum and cerebrum.
- It is conventional to consider that disequilibrium which is vestibular in origin will be caused by disorders in either the peripheral or central systems. On most occasions this is not the case, as the majority of pathological processes affect both the peripheral and central vestibular systems.
- Disorders of the visual system are uncommon and relatively easy to identify. For practical purposes they can be discounted.
- In the majority of individuals with disequilibrium, a definite pathology will not be identified.

- As such the majority will have a syndrome/symptom complex ascribed to them.
- Syndrome/symptom complexes are identified from the patient's history.
- The clinical examination will vary depending on the history and will exclude in most individuals the probability of serious central pathology.
- The majority of patients do not require sophisticated investigations.
- Caloric testing detects hypofunction in the peripheral vestibular system.
- Not all peripheral syndromes/diseases are associated with hypofunction on caloric testing.
- Caloric testing does not attempt to arrive at a specific diagnosis of the aetiology of disequilibrium.
- Electronystagmography allows eye movements to be recorded with the eyes shut and to be mathematically analysed. Its interpretation, to give additional diagnostic information, is difficult and mainly of interest to the neuro-otologist.
- In the majority of patients the disequilibrium will settle with time, so reassurance is the mainstay of management until this occurs.
- Medication is by no means necessary in all patients and this applies especially to the elderly in whom it can make matters worse.
- No one drug would appear to be of greater efficacy than any other in controlling acute symptoms or in the prevention of recurrent episodes.

• Surgery for vertigo, such as endolymphatic sac decompression, is yet to be proven to be of greater value than placebo operations.

• The reasons for this are that surgery of any type has a considerable placebo effect and the disequilibrium in most individuals will resolve with time anyway.

• For the difficult-to-manage patient a placebo operation should not be discounted.

• Alternatively, labyrinthectomy or vestibular nerve section can be carried out but the former destroys residual hearing and the latter is an intracranial operation.

Further reading

Benyon, G.J. (1997). A review of management of benign paroxysmal positional vertigo by exercise therapy and by repositioning manoeuvres. *British Journal of Audiology*, **31**, 11–26.

Cawthorne, T.E. and Cooksey, C. (1997). Cawthorne–Cooksey regime of head exercises. In *Otology*, Vol. 3, Appendix 12.1, p. 3/12/27, Scott-Brown's Otolaryngology, 6th Edition. Butterworth-Heinemann, Oxford.

Commins, D.J. and Nedzelski, J.M. (1996). Current diagnostics and office practice. Topical drugs in the treatment of Ménière's disease. *Current Opinion in Otolaryngology & Head and Neck Surgery*, **4**, 319–323.

Shepard, N.T. and Telian, S.A. (1996). *Practical Management of the Balance Disorder Patient*. Singular Publishing Group, San Diego, CA.

Appendix I

Value of investigations

Sensitivity (true-positive rate or hit rate)

Sensitivity is the percentage of patients with a condition that are correctly identified by a test. A sensitivity of 100 per cent is the target for a test, i.e. all the patients with a condition are correctly identified.

Specificity (true-negative rate)

Specificity is the percentage of patients who do not have a condition that are correctly categorized by the test. A specificity of 100 per cent is the target for a test, i.e. all the patients that do not have a condition are correctly identified.

False-negative rate

This is the percentage of patients with a condition that are not identified by a test. This rate is calculated by subtracting the sensitivity of a test from 100 per cent.

False-alarm rate

This is the percentage of patients that do not have a condition that are incorrectly categorized as having the condition by the test. The rate is calculated by subtracting the specificity of the test from 100 per cent.

Example 1
Straight X-rays of the internal auditory canal have a sensitivity of 70 per cent and a specificity of 80 per cent in detecting acoustic neuromas.

- Of 100 patients with an acoustic neuroma, 70 will be identified by X-ray and 30 will be missed by X-ray.
- Of 100 patients that do not have an acoustic neuroma, 80 will be identified as not having an acoustic neuroma and 20 will be falsely diagnosed as having an acoustic neuroma.

	Acoustic neuroma	No acoustic neuroma	Total
X-ray +ve	70	20	90
X-ray −ve	30	80	110
Total	100	100	200

	Sensitivity	Specificity
	$\dfrac{70}{70 + 30}$	$\dfrac{80}{80 + 20}$
	70%	80%

Predictive values

In clinical practice, the usefulness of a test depends on more than sensitivity and specificity. This is because the incidence of a disease varies depending on the situation in which a test is applied. Thus, in Example 2, taking the incidence as 5 per cent of patients with an asymmetric sensorineural hearing impairment, in an ENT clinic of 200 patients screened, 10 will have an acoustic neuroma and 190 will not. On the other hand, in a tertiary referral clinic, the incidence of acoustic neuromas will be considerably greater, say 50 per cent. The value of straight X-rays will be different in each clinic. It is thus necessary to work out the positive and negative predictive values of a test for each situation, and this involves knowing the incidence of the condition in the population being tested.

Thus in Example 3, in a tertiary referral clinic when the incidence of acoustic neuroma is 50 per cent, the predictive value of a positive straight X-ray is 78 per cent, compared with 16 per cent in an ENT clinic, just because the incidence of acoustic neuromas is higher at the tertiary clinic.

Example 2
In the average ENT clinic:

	Acoustic neuroma	No acoustic neuroma	Total
X-ray +ve	7	38	45
X-ray −ve	3	152	155
Total	10	190	200

Predictive value of +ve test: $\dfrac{7}{45} = 16\%$

Predictive value of −ve test: $\dfrac{152}{155} = 98\%$

Sensitivity:
$\dfrac{7}{10}$
70%

Specificity:
$\dfrac{152}{190}$
80%

Hence in the ENT clinic, far more patients will have a false-positive X-ray of an acoustic neuroma than will have an actual tumour (38 compared with 7). Though the predictive value of a negative test appears high at 98 per cent, 3 out of the 10 patients with an acoustic neuroma will have a negative X-ray.

Example 3
In the tertiary referral clinic:

	Acoustic neuroma	No acoustic neuroma	Total
X-ray +ve	70	20	90
X-ray −ve	30	80	110
Total	100	100	200

Predictive value of +ve test: $\dfrac{70}{90} = 78\%$

Predictive value of −ve test: $\dfrac{80}{110} = 73\%$

Sensitivity:
$\dfrac{70}{100}$
70%

Specificity:
$\dfrac{80}{100}$
80%

Combining the results of two tests

The naive might think that two tests are better than one. Unfortunately this is not the case. There are two ways in which the two tests can be analysed: (1) at least one test has to be positive; or (2) both tests have to be positive. The problem with the first approach is that the reasons why a patient passes or fails a test are not necessarily the same for each test. The sensitivity may improve and specificity get worse. With the second approach of requiring two positive tests, though the specificity is improved the sensitivity deteriorates (*Table AI.1*). An alternative method is sequential testing. In this method, the second test is only done if the first test is positive. The criterion is then two positive tests. This increases the specificity but reduces the sensitivity.

Table AI.1 The potential hit and false-negative rates in individuals being screened using brain stem electric response audiometry and acoustic reflexes as examples

	Sensitivity (%)	*Specificity* (%)
Test battery:		
Loose criterion (1 positive test)	95–100	50–70
Strict criterion (2 positive tests)	80–85	80–100
Sequential battery:		
Strict criterion (2 positive tests)	81	94

Appendix II

Methods of pure tone audiometry[*]

General points

Instructions to patient

- Indicate as soon as you hear the tone and for as long as you continue to hear it.
- No matter how faint the tones are or in which ear they are heard, respond when you hear them.

Patient's response

- Absent if no response for whole duration of signal.

Test signal

- On for 1–3 second burst.
- Randomly vary durations of both tones and intervals.

Order of test

(1) Test the better hearing ear first.
(2) 1, 2, (3), 4, (6), 8, 0.5, 0.25 kHz, and then retest 1 kHz.
(3) 1, 2, (3), 4, (6), 8, 0.5, 0.25 kHz in the other ear.

*Abbreviated version of British Society of Audiology and British Association of Otolaryngologists and Head and Neck Surgeons recommendations.

Familiarization

- A 3 second tone at estimated threshold +30 dB.
- If not heard, increase in 20 dB steps until heard.
- Check correct manner of response.

Test method A

- Drop in 10 dB steps until not heard.
- Raise in 5 dB steps until heard.
- Repeat as required, down in 10 dB steps, up in 5 dB steps.
- Threshold is lowest level at which 50 per cent or more of ascending signals are heard, with minimum of two responses at that level.

Test method B

- Drop in 10 dB steps until not heard.
- When not heard, present two or three more tones at that level.
- (a) If 'heard' (at least two responses out of four) lower lever by 5 dB, or
- (b) If 'not heard' (one or no responses out of four) raise level by 5 dB.
- Repeat stages (a) or (b), as far as necessary.
- Threshold is lowest level 'heard'.

Symbols

○   Right air conduction
●   Right air conduction, false not masked
     threshold
×   Left air conduction
⊻   Left air conduction, false not masked
     threshold
Δ   Bone conduction, not masked

[Right bone conduction, masked
]   Left bone conduction, masked

↘ with any symbol indicates that the threshold is poorer at that level but it cannot be determined because of the limited output in that mode of presentation of the audiometer being used.

Appendix III

Examples of masking in pure tone audiometry

The seven examples illustrate in sequential stages the assessment of the pure tone threshold at a single frequency. The symbols are those internationally recognized and detailed in Appendix II.

Example 1

1. No further testing is required as no air-bone (a–b) gap is present in either ear. The unmasked bone conduction (b–c) applies to both ears.

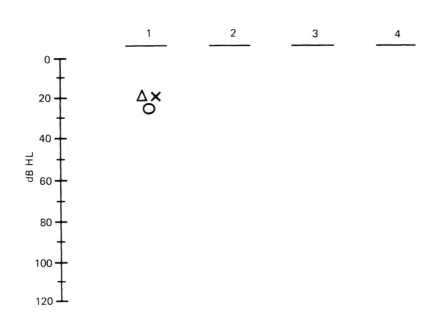

Example 2

1. Potential a–b gap right.
   Right b–c requires to be reassessed with masking of the left ear.

2. No a–b gap in either ear.
   Not masked b–c applies to left ear.
   No need to reassess right air conduction (a–c) as difference between right a–c and left b–c is less than 40 dB.
   Test complete.

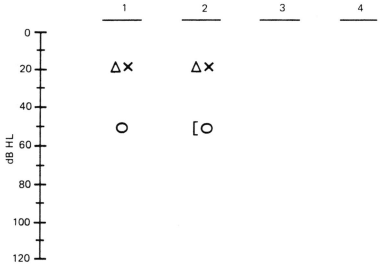

Example 3

1. Potential a–b gap in one or both ears.
   Either right or left ear b–c can be assessed with masking of the other ear. Right ear is chosen to be assessed with masking of the left ear.

2. No a–b gap right.
   Not masked b–c must apply to left.
   Test complete.

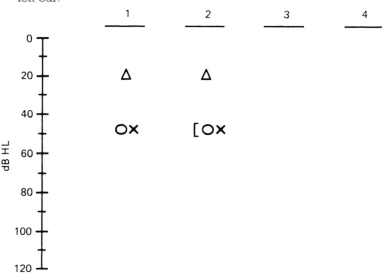

Example 4

1. Potential a–b gap in one or both ears. Either right or left ear b–c can be assessed with masking of the other ear. Right ear is chosen to be assessed with masking of the left ear.

2. Right a–b gap. Left b–c requires to be assessed with masking of right.

3. Bilateral a–b gaps. The a–c in neither ear is greater than b–c in other ear by 40 dB so there is no need to reassess the a–c thresholds. Test complete.

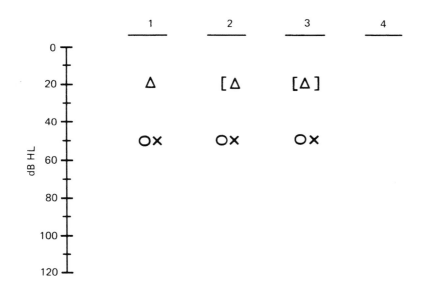

Example 5

1. Potential a–b gap in one or both ears. Either right or left ear b–c can be assessed with masking of the other ear. Right ear is chosen to be assessed with masking of the left ear.

2. Right a–b gap. Left b–c requires to be assessed with masking of right.

3. Right a–b gap. No a–b gap left. Test complete.

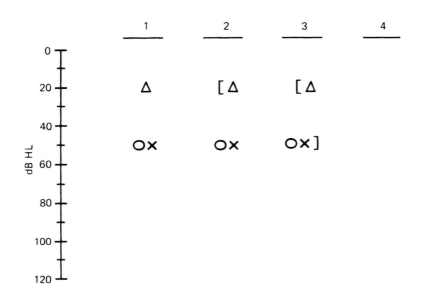

Example 6

1. Potential a–b gap in one or both ears. Either right or left ear b–c can be assessed with masking of the other ear. Right ear is chosen to be assessed with masking of the left ear.

2. Right a–b gap. Left b–c requires to be assessed with masking of right.
3. As the difference between left a–c and right b–c is 40 dB the left a–c requires to be reassessed with masking of the right ear.
4. Left a–c when reassessed with masking of the right ear is 100 dB. Test complete.

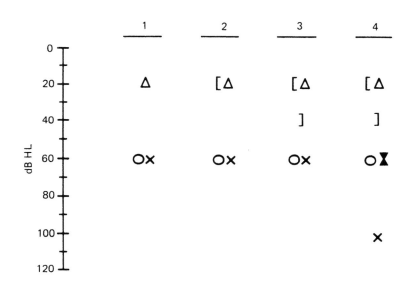

Example 7

1. Potential a–b gap right.
   Right b–c requires to be reassessed with masking of the left ear.
2. Right b–c outside upper range of output of b–c vibrator of audiometer.
   Right a–c requires reassessment with masking of the left as there is a 40 dB difference between apparent right a–c and left b–c.
3. Right a–c outside upper range of output of a–c of audiometer.
   Dead right ear.
   Test complete.

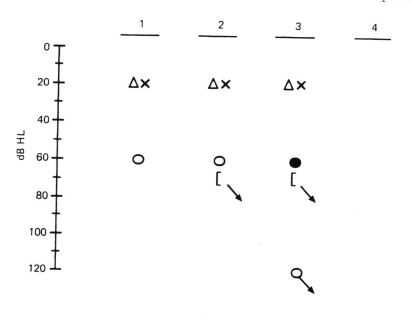

Appendix IV

Acoustic impedance

Acoustic impedance is being increasingly used in otology, one of its main advantages being that the only requirement made of the patient is that they remain comparatively still during the test. This appendix concentrates on the practical aspects of acoustic impedance. Its clinical usefulness is discussed in the various contexts in which it can be used.

The scientific basis of acoustic impedance is complicated but, thankfully, it is not necessary for the otologist to understand it to interpret the results. For those interested it has been well explained elsewhere (Lutman, 1986; Gelfand, 1997a). All that needs to be known initially is that, in clinical use, acoustic impedance can be subdivided into tympanometry and acoustic reflexes.

Tympanometry

All machines, whether portable or not, have an ear-piece with three channels which is inserted into the test ear (*Figure AIV.1*). One channel introduces sound into the external auditory canal, the second has a microphone which records the sound level within the external auditory canal and the third allows the pressure in the external canal to be varied. When the ear-piece is in the canal and the tympanic membrane is intact, the canal acts as a rigid tube with a compliant end. Sound intro-duced into this cavity will be absorbed to a degree dependent on the ability of the tympanic membrane and the ossicular chain to transfer sound to the inner ear. The amount of sound that is absorbed depends on the compliance of the middle ear system and can be calculated by measuring the resultant sound level in the canal. (In practice the sound level in the canal is held constant and the amount of energy required to hold it constant is measured.)

The compliance is primarily related to the stiffness of the tympanic membrane which can be affected by many factors including its own mobility, the pressure differential between the middle ear and the canal, and the state of the ossicular chain, the last factor having only a minor influence. It is possible to vary the canal pressure via one of the channels in the ear-piece. The actual pressure that can be achieved varies depending on the machine but usually ranges from -400 to $+200$ deca-Pascals (daPa) which is often expressed as millimetres of water pressure (mmH_2O) as this is more meaningful to clinicians. The tympanic membrane will be most compliant when the external canal pressure is the same as that in the middle ear. So by varying the pressure in the canal and monitoring the compliance, it is possible to estimate the middle ear pressure. When the canal pressure is altered to ~ 200 mmH_2O above or below middle ear

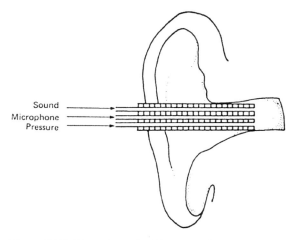

Figure AIV.1 Three channels of the ear probe

pressure the tympanic membrane will become relatively stiff. The canal then approximates to a hard-walled cavity which reflects all the sound put into it. This minimum compliance is subtracted from the maximum compliance to give the combined compliance of the tympanic membrane and ossicular chain.

The compliance of the tympanic membrane and ossicular chain is often erroneously thought to be the same as its degree of mobility as assessed by pneumatic otoscopy. They measure different but comparable aspects of function.

Most otologists do not take any particular notice of the compliance values but look at the tympanogram to decide which one of three shapes it most resembles (*Figure AIV.2* and *Table 13.1*, p. 138). An alternative method is to say whether the tympanogram is peaked or non-peaked and to quote the pressure at which it is peaked.

Type A

This is a peaked tympanogram within the normal middle ear pressure range −99 to +200 mmH$_2$O. It is suggested to occur in normal ears, and with otosclerosis and ossicular discontinuity.

Type C

This type shows a definite peak in the compliance with negative pressure less than −100 mmH$_2$O. It is suggested to occur in

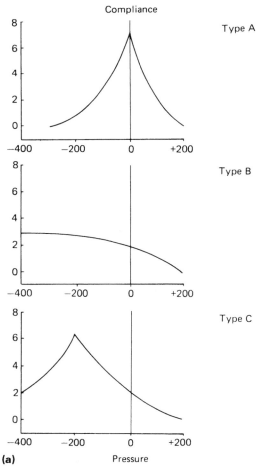

(a)

Figure AIV.2 Classification of tympanogram shapes (after Jerger, 1970)

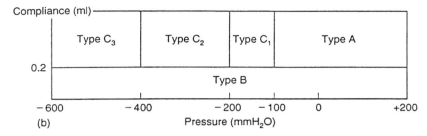

Figure AIV.2 (*continued*)

those with Eustachian tube dysfunction and perhaps in those with otitis media with effusion. Type C tympanograms can be subdivided depending on the pressure of the peak: C_1 −100 to −199; C_2 −200 to −399; C_3 −400 to −600 mmH$_2$O. The more negative the peak pressure, the more likely is the diagnosis of otitis media with effusion.

Type B

Here there is no obvious peak to the compliance over the pressure range of the machine. Most machines do not go down as far as −600 mmH$_2$O. Hence on most machines a type C_3 would be classified as a type B. It is suggested to occur in otitis media with effusion.

Practical considerations

One of the most frequent complaints that inexperienced technicians have regarding tympanometry is that it is difficult to obtain a seal. It should be possible to obtain a seal in more than 95 per cent of ears if the correct technique is used. As in most things, the first attempt usually has the best chance of success. The size of the ear canal should be estimated by examination and an appropriately sized probe tip selected. Though it may be initially uncomfortable for the patient the tip should be inserted with a little force and a slight twist. If this is done there will be few failures.

Clinical value of tympanometry

Tympanometry is mainly used to diagnose otitis media with effusion (see p. 138). In doing

this the shape of the tympanogram is most frequently used. The pressure at which the tympanogram peaks is considered to accurately reflect the actual middle ear pressure. Unfortunately this is not so as the volume of the middle ear and mastoid air space also has an influence (Gaihede, 1998). Because of the range of compliance in normal ears, the procedure is not of value in the diagnosis of otosclerosis or ossicular discontinuity.

Acoustic reflexes

If sound of sufficient intensity is introduced into a normal ear, reflex contraction of the stapedius muscle occurs in both ears provided the facial nerve and brain stem are functioning normally. These contractions result in a small change in the compliance of the middle ear and a contralateral or ipsilateral reflex is then said to be present depending on which ear was stimulated by the sound (*Figure AIV.3*). Testing for acoustic reflexes presupposes that the facial nerve is normal. This is usually assumed to be the case if the patient has no obvious palsy or a history of one in the past.

Method

The equipment is the same as that used for tympanometry, the only addition being a monaural head-set which delivers the sound to the non-probe ear when contralateral reflexes are being tested. Most modern machines have this facility with the exception of some of the semi-automatic machines which can only stimulate ipsilateral reflexes.

Reflexes can be stimulated using pure tones

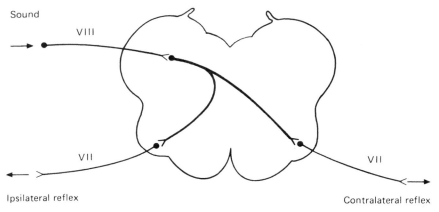

Sound

VIII

VII

Ipsilateral reflex

VII

Contralateral reflex

Figure AIV.3 Acoustic reflex pathways

or with a wide- or narrow-band noise. It is more usual to test with pure tones at 0.5, 1, 2 and 4 kHz and, in order to increase the test's reliability, at least two tones should be tested. A tympanogram is initially obtained from which the middle ear pressure is estimated and reflex testing is thereafter carried out at this pressure. The sound is delivered to the ear to be stimulated via the headphone for contralateral reflexes and via the probe for ipsilateral reflexes. Testing for a reflex commences at a reasonable level above the pure tone threshold, usually about 80 dB HL, and the compliance needle is observed for a deflection which indicates a present reflex. Alternatively the reflexes can be recorded on a plotter. If a reflex is not elicited the sound level is increased until a reflex is obtained, the maximum output of most machines being ∼ 120 dB SPL.

It is usual to begin by testing for contralateral reflexes and, if these are not obtained, to progress to ipsilateral stimulation. In order to elicit a contralateral reflex in a normal ear, the level of the sound stimulus has to be considerably above that of the pure tone threshold at that frequency in the stimulated ear. In the majority (95 per cent) of individuals whose pure tone thresholds are less than 25 dB, the reflex thresholds will be between 70 and 100 dB above their pure tone threshold at that frequency (*Figure AIV.4*). As the maximum output of most machines is 120 dB one would not expect to elicit a reflex if the threshold in the stimulated ear was greater than 45 dB HL but for practical purposes, because of recruit-

ment, this figure can be increased to 55 dB HL (*Figure AIV.5*).

Data are surprisingly lacking regarding ipsilateral stimulation but it is generally considered to be less reliable for technical reasons than contralateral stimulation. Until data are available it would seem reasonable to apply the same rules as for contralateral stimulation.

Interpretation of results

The results can be used in two ways. The presence or absence of a reflex can be used to predict the likelihood of there being a conductive defect in the probe ear. Whether the probe ear is recruiting can be assessed by the amount the reflex threshold is above the pure tone threshold at that frequency. Normally the reflex thresholds will be at least 70 dB above the pure tone threshold but the level of this can vary considerably (*Figure AIV.4*). In recruiting ears the difference is not so marked and can be as low as 10 dB. The advantage of acoustic reflex tests in assessing recruitment is that they do not require the patient's co-operation and they can be performed irrespective of whether there is an impairment in the other ear or not. Their disadvantage is that they require a present reflex.

It is also possible to detect abnormal adaptation (i.e. acoustic reflex decay which is not necessarily the same as tone decay) by the duration that a reflex lasts. This is best recorded by a plotter and normally a reflex should last for at least 10 seconds before decaying to 50 per

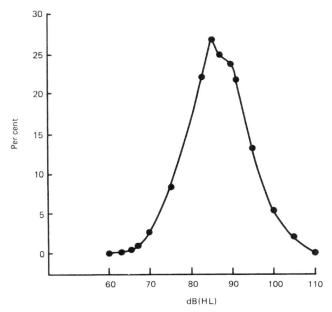

Figure AIV.4 Contralateral reflex thresholds in normal ears (after Jerger *et al.*, 1972)

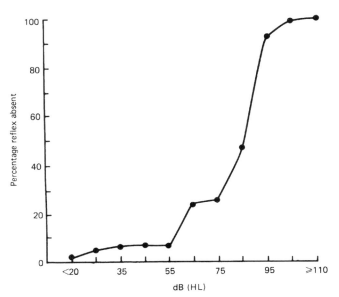

Figure AIV.5 Percentage reflexes present related to the pure tone average in the contralateral, sound stimulated ear (after Jerger *et al.*, 1972)

cent of its starting value. Indeed acoustic reflexes would appear to be one of the better audiometric tests for doing this, with a sensitivity for detection of retrocochlear pathology of ~ 85 per cent in individuals who are able to be tested. The specificity is also reasonably low at ~ 20 per cent.

Further reading

Gelfand, S.A. (1977). Acoustic immitance assessment. In *Essentials of Audiology*, Chap. 7. Thieme Verlag, New York.

Jerger, J. and Northern, J.L. (1980). *Clinical Impedance Audiometry*, 2nd Edition. American Electromedics Corporation, Acton, MA.

Appendix V

Speech audiometry

Over the years many different tests have been used which utilize the spoken word. The tests vary in detail but essentially the speech can be presented either monaurally or binaurally, and either free-field or over headphones. The speech can be words or sentences, sense or nonsense, with or without competing noise and with or without an associated visual presentation. The method of scoring can be based on percentages correct or based on the level of the signal required to achieve a set score. Which combination is used depends on what is being assessed. For example, a different combination might be used to assess hearing impairment than the combination used to assess disability.

In clinical practice the term 'speech audiometry' is reserved for monaural tests presented in quiet conditions over headphones and scored as the percentage correct at various sound intensities. This appendix deals with the practical aspects of this type of speech audiometry and whether this disability is reduced by surgery or a hearing aid.

Test method

In conventional speech audiometry, words are used in preference to sentences because of the greater redundancy of information in the latter. In addition, if a test list is going to be used on several occasions it is better that the subject's ability to remember the list is minimal. This is less likely to occur with words than it is with sentences. On any one test occasion several lists of words of equal difficulty and phonetic balance must be available to test the patient at different sound levels. Considerable effort has gone into achieving this and, in the United Kingdom, Boothroyd's, Fry's and the MRC lists are those most commonly used. In the USA, the CID and the Harvard lists are preferred.

The word lists are recorded on tape and presented via a normal audiometer to the patient monaurally over headphones and at various sound levels. The use of a live voice is to be deprecated because of the impossibility of maintaining a steady sound level.

As speech audiometry is a suprathreshold test, the normal rules of masking do not apply. It must be assumed that the other ear might hear the speech irrespective of the sound level. Masking of the non-test ear with broad band noise is therefore required on all occasions. The masking levels that are used can be calculated from a formula that takes into account the degree of air-conduction symmetry, any air–bone gap and the calibration values of the machine (Coles and Priede, 1977).

The patient is asked to repeat back the words as accurately as possible and the percentage of words or phonemes (i.e. parts of words) correctly repeated, is plotted on a graph against sound pressure level. This is compared with the calibration graph (*Figure AV.1*) for that particular machine which will have been obtained by testing otologically normal individuals on that machine, using the same tapes and test environment. It is essential to make this comparison because this is the only way that speech audiometry can be calibrated, the readings of the sound pressure level on the dial being different for each machine, tape and test environment.

From the patient's speech audiogram (speech discrimination curve, performance intensity [PI] curve) several values can be read off. Unfortunately different terms are used for these values in different centres which can give rise to confusion.

Optimal discrimination score (ODS) or maximum discrimination score

This is the highest score that can be achieved by the patient, no matter how loud the volume. Normally a patient's optimal discrimination score (ODS) would be expected to be no more than 30 dB above their pure tone average and, as such, individuals with a pure tone average of greater than 70 dB HL, might not achieve their potential ODS because the maximum output of most machines is ~ 100 dB dial units (*Figure AV.2*).

When a short word list (e.g. 10 words) is used, a test/retest error of 10 per cent has to be allowed for, because it is relatively easy to miss one word due to inattention.

Half peak level elevation (HPLE)

The half peak level (HPL) is the dB level at which, by interpolation from the speech graph, the individual would be expected to achieve half their ODS. As the dB dial output of each machine is different, the HPL by itself is of limited value. The half peak level elevation (HPLE) is a more relevant measure. This is the dB level at which the patient achieves half their ODS in comparison with the level at which normal individuals achieve 50 per cent. So for an individual with an ODS of 70 per cent, the HPLE is the dial reading at which they achieve a 35 per cent score minus the dial reading at which a normal individual achieves 50 per cent. Thus, in *Figure AV.3*, the ODS is 70 per cent and the half ODS is therefore 35 per cent. From the patient's graph, the level at which they would be expected to achieve a score of 35 per cent is ~ 54 dB. (It is not necessary to have actually tested the patient at this point to calculate the HPL.) By reference to the calibration graph for that machine (*Figure AV.1*) the HPL of a normal individual would be 15 dB. The patient's HPLE is 54 − 15 = 39 dB.

The advantage of the HPLE is that it can be calculated for an individual whose ODS is less than 50 per cent.

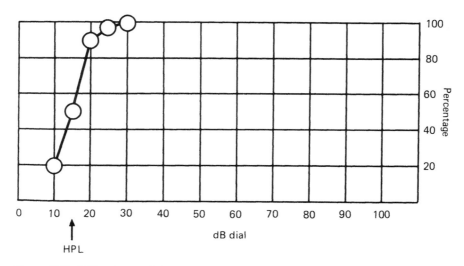

Figure AV.1 Calibration graph for a particular audiometer, tape and environment

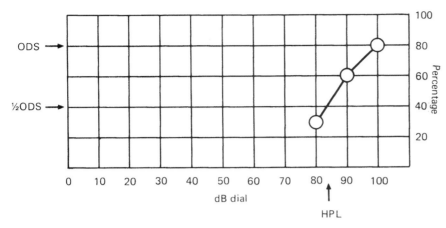

Figure AV.2 ODS of 80 per cent, to be interpreted with caution as it is at the maximum output of this machine

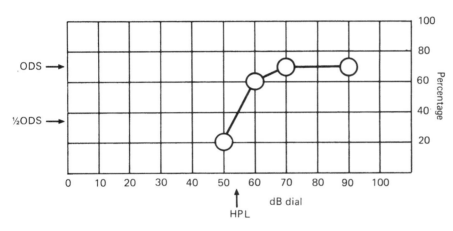

Figure AV.3

Speech reception threshold (SRT)

This is the SPL at which the patient achieves a 50 per cent score. The SRT is perhaps a less valuable measure than the HPLE because in a clinic population 38 per cent of patients do not achieve an ODS of 50 per cent in their *poorer* hearing ear (Glasgow Royal Infirmary clinic data).

Speech audiogram (curve) shape

There are two basic shapes to be recognized. The 'normal' shape is where the speech discrimination peaks and then remains the same with increasing SPLs (*Figure AV.3*). A 'roll-over' shape is where the speech discrimination

score deteriorates with increasing SPLs after the ODS has been reached (*Figure AV.4*).

Speech detection threshold

This measure is only mentioned to avoid confusion when reading the literature. It is the level at which a patient detects but cannot necessarily repeat any of the words. The speech detection threshold gives no additional information to that obtained from a pure tone audiogram.

Clinical value

In otology there are five main aspects that are normally assessed: (i) whether there is a hear-

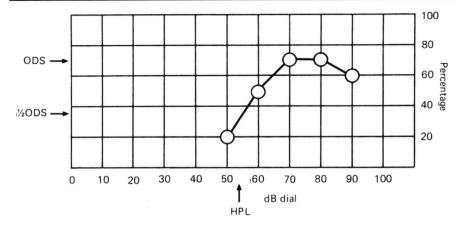

Figure AV.4 'Roll-over' curve

ing impairment and if so (ii) where it is, (iii) what has caused it, (iv) what disability it has given rise to and (v) whether this disability is reduced by surgery or a hearing aid. Speech audiometry has been used to evaluate all of these aspects but it is most frequently used to assess a hearing impairment and the resultant disability.

Assessment of hearing impairment

Pure tone audiometry assesses the threshold of detection of pure tones. It does not assess the ability to differentiate at suprathreshold levels between sounds of different frequencies, loudness and timing. Speech audiometry measures a combination of these and is the only test that is currently available in most clinics which will do this. Speech audiometry has many defects but, in particular, a lack of precision because of the considerable amount of redundant information present in a word which it is not necessary to hear in order to identify it. Despite this, speech audiometry is considered superior to pure tone audiometry as a method of assessing the hearing.

The evidence that this is so can be seen in an analysis of data available from patients attending on audiology clinic. Accepting that there might be a 10 per cent error in the scores because of test errors, 62 per cent of clinic patients do not achieve an ODS of 90 per cent in their better ear no matter how loud the volume is turned up (*Figure AV.5*, Glasgow Royal Infirmary clinic data). In 18 per cent of patients the ODS is 50 per cent or less in their better ear. If the pure tone thresholds (*Figure AV.6*) were all that were to have been available, it is unlikely that most of these poor scores would have been suspected. At present it is not known where the primary pathology is that has given rise to these poor scores but there are major implications regarding disability and the likelihood of success in management.

Assessment of disability

There are many different types of situation where a patient may have a disability because of their hearing impairment. Asking patients how much trouble they have in a specific situation is the best means, at present, of assessing their disability but it would be better if disability tests were available. Until this occurs it will be up to the otologist to extract what information he can from the results that are available to him. More information is available about disability from the HPLE or the ODS in the better ear than from the pure tone average.

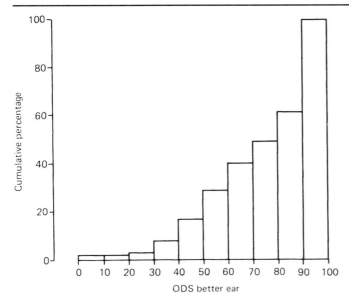

Figure AV.5 Cumulative distribution of ODS in the better ear of a clinic population (Glasgow Royal Infirmary clinic data)

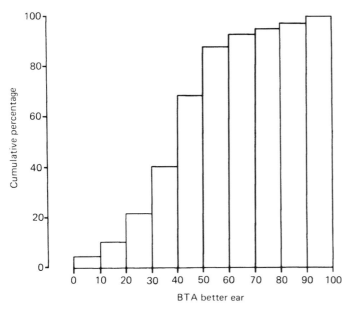

Figure AV.6 Cumulative distribution of the best two pure tone averages in the better ear of a clinic population (Glasgow Royal Infirmary clinic data). BTA = best two average

■ Conclusions

• Monaural speech audiometry gives a wider appraisal of a patient's hearing than pure tone audiometry.

• Though speech discrimination impairments can be easily detected, it is not possible to attribute them to a specific pathological process or to decide what auditory function is at fault.

• Speech audiometry may give a better indication of disability than the pure tone audiogram.

Appendix VI

Stenger test

Tuning fork test

The Stenger test is used to detect a feigned, asymmetric hearing impairment when in fact the hearing in the two ears is similar. Two identical tuning forks are required and the basis of the test is that when sounds of the same frequency are presented at different intensities to both ears, it will only be heard in the ear with the stronger sensation level.

The test is carried out from behind the patient, to make sure that they do not see what is being done. An activated fork is presented to the good ear and will be reported to be heard (*Figure AVI.1*). It is then presented to the feigned or truly bad ear and will be reported not to be heard. The two forks are then equally activated and placed equidistant, about 1 foot from each ear. Both feigning and genuine patients will report hearing it in their good ear. The fork beside the 'bad' ear is gradually moved closer to it. In a true unilateral loss the patient will continue to hear the sound in the good ear and will say so. In a feigned asymmetric loss, the sound will be heard in the 'bad' ear because of the stronger sensation level. As they cannot admit to this, they have to state that they cannot hear the sound in either ear and this is obviously incorrect.

No figures appear to be available on the effectiveness of the Stenger test in identifying asymmetric exaggerated thresholds. In prac-

tice it is difficult to activate two tuning forks equally.

Audiometric test

In an individual who is exaggerating the hearing impairment in one ear, the audiometric Stenger test can be used to ascertain what the pure tone thresholds are likely to be. The test is not applicable when the thresholds in both ears are being exaggerated and it relies upon accurate thresholds being available for the other ear. The test is best explained by reference to *Table VI.1*.

Let us take an example where the proffered thresholds at a specific frequency are 5 dB HL in the left and 50 dB HL in the right ear. A signal of 5 dB above the threshold is presented to the left ear (at 10 dB) and kept there at each subsequent step in the test. In the ear with the exaggerated thresholds the signal is progressively reduced in 5 dB steps starting at the proffered thresholds. On each occasion the patient is asked to respond when a tone is heard, no matter in which ear it is heard. In the example given the patient will hear the 45 dB signal in the right ear but as they are feigning their thresholds they will be unwilling to admit it. The signal being presented to the right ear is gradually reduced in 5 dB steps until the point is reached when the patient actually

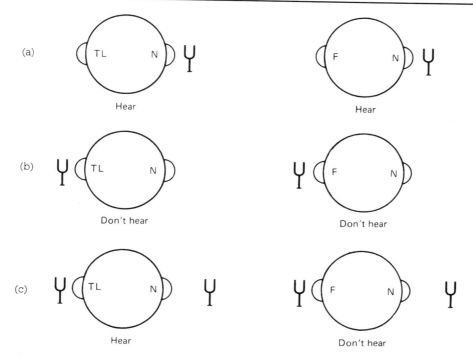

(a)

Hear   Hear

(b)

Don't hear   Don't hear

(c)

Hear   Don't hear

Figure AVI.1 Likely response to the Stenger test of patients who have a true loss (TL) or a false loss (F) in one ear. The hearing in the other ear is normal (N). The position of the tuning fork symbol indicates its relative distance from the ear

hears the 10 dB signal in their left ear and admits to hearing it. The level at which the patient changes from stating that they hear nothing to the level at which they hear it in the good ear indicates the likely threshold in the ear with the exaggerated loss. In this instance the true threshold in the right ear is between 25 and 30 dB HL at the frequency being tested.

Table VI.1 Audiometric Stenger test sequence

Presentation order	Level of presentation		Patient response
	Left	Right	
1	10	45	Don't hear
2	10	40	Don't hear
3	10	35	Don't hear
4	10	30	? Hear in left ear
5	10	25	Hear in left ear

Appendix VII

Electric response audiometry

Background

When an ear is stimulated by sound, the hair cells are activated and this results in electric stimuli which travel along the auditory nerve to the cochlear nuclei in the brain stem on both sides, thence to the superior olivary complex, to the nucleus of the lateral lemniscus, to the inferior colliculus, to the medial geniculate body and finally to the cerebral auditory cortex. It is possible to detect these auditory responses in any part of the pathway using standard electroencephalographic (EEG) techniques and recording at the appropriate time after the stimulus.

The practical problem is how to separate out the auditory responses from other neural activity. This is done by presenting multiple auditory signals and averaging the responses with a computer so that the auditory responses are enhanced and the other electrical signals are cancelled out. The technique is called electric response audiometry (ERA) and auditory evoked potentials (AEP) are what is recorded. The object is to get both a readable and an accurate response. More readable responses are achieved by increasing the number of stimuli especially when the responses are small. Greater accuracy is achieved by increasing the number of stimuli and repeating the assessment when at threshold levels. Lack of time is a limiting factor in ERA but it is better

spent gaining two reliable thresholds rather than several unreliable ones.

These responses can be picked up with electrodes placed anywhere on the head, but practical experience has shown that a vertex electrode along with an earth electrode on the mastoid or ear lobe is the best combination. The obvious exception to this is electrocochleography which is recorded from the middle ear promontory via a transtympanic electrode or by an electrode in the external auditory canal near the tympanic membrane. Because the electrode is close to the auditory nerve this technique requires fewer auditory signals to be presented for a satisfactory response to be averaged and does not require masking.

The following introductory comments attempt to rectify some incorrect impressions that some might have rather than to denigrate the technique.

- ERA is *not* an objective test of hearing. It is true that the patient's active co-operation is not required and, as such, it is extensively used in medico-legal work and in the assessment of difficult-to-test children. Though equipment is being increasingly automated, what in general is produced are lots of squiggly lines which someone has to interpret. It is here that the method stops being objective and becomes subjective, any small peak or dip in the squiggle being interpretable as a response. Correspondingly, interpreting the tracing is only for the experienced who have tested many different types of patients.

- The number of patients in any ORL practice who need to have their thresholds of hearing assessed by ERA is small. Assessment by standard audiological methods is always preferable because these are quicker, cheaper and more accurate.

- In a normal ORL clinic there will be patients who need to be screened to exclude an acoustic neuroma but the audiometric or radiographic test which is used will depend considerably on the expertise available. In the hands of experts, ERA has a high sensitivity but it cannot be advocated as a screening test in departments where there is limited expertise. This is because the sensitivity and specificity are likely to be poorer due to misinterpreting peaks in the trace when calculating latencies.

- The thresholds obtained by ERA are not as accurate as some might think. Calibration errors can be present as the equipment has to be calibrated on normal individuals and thereafter checked regularly. As in any other form of audiometry, over- or undermasking can easily occur and indeed is more likely because the masking levels often have to be arbitrarily chosen.

- Finally, though the mean ERA thresholds may correspond fairly well to the mean pure tone thresholds in a series of patients, there can be considerable difference between the two thresholds in a specific patient. In a slow vertex electrical response, the difference at an individual frequency can be as great as 35 dB (Davis, 1984; Coles and Mason, 1984; see *Table 8.2*, p. 77) though this will be reduced if several frequencies are averaged.

Techniques

The average otologist does not need to have a detailed knowledge of the techniques or be able to interpret the results, unless they wish to carry out ERA themselves, when they would be advised to learn under supervision rather than by trial and error. On the other hand, all otologists should understand the advantages and disadvantages of the three main types of ERA so that the appropriate test can be requested when they have a patient in whom conventional audiometry has failed.

As with any audiometric technique, testing ought to be carried out in a sound-proofed environment. In addition, artefacts can be caused by electrical interference, particularly if X-ray and other electrical equipment is being used nearby.

It is a common mistake to think that ERA machines come calibrated and the dB settings on the stimulus and masking sound dials are hearing levels. Each of the sound and masking signals has to be biologically calibrated on normally hearing individuals as there are no standards to enable this to be done otherwise at present.

In practical terms three main types of response are recorded, the difference between them being the time (latency) after the auditory stimuli when they occur rather than the siting of the electrodes:

- the electrocochleogram (ECochG);
- the auditory brain stem response (ABR);
- the cortical evoked potentials.

Several different sound stimuli can be used to initiate a response and which is used depends on what is being assessed by which method. A click has a sharp on/off time with a known phase. In theory clicks are broad-band sounds but, in practice, they tend to be centred on 3 kHz because of the frequency response of the earphone. They can also be filtered to give a click at any desired frequency. A tone pip is a segment of a sinusoidal tone and its phase can be controlled.

In all three methods, thresholds are determined by progressively decreasing the sound level of the stimulus until no response can be detected. This is not as easy as it might seem because as the sound intensity decreases, the latency of the response increases and this can make it difficult to be sure whether there is a response or not. It is at this point that the method stops being objective and becomes subjective. To minimize the effect of observer interpretation, at least three repetitions at each level are performed and a positive response is only considered to be present if there is an apparent response in two out of the three replications.

Masking of the non-test ear is as essential in

ERA as it is in other forms of audiometry, the exception being ECochG where the recording is made directly from the test ear. Masking is delivered via a headphone and when the true threshold in the non-test ear is known, the appropriate masking level can be calculated. When it is not known, the appropriate level is guessed at.

Neuro-otological pathology is detected primarily by an increase in the latency of the V wave response compared with normal. In addition, abnormal variations in the amplitude of the response can be helpful.

Each of the techniques has its advantages and its disadvantages, its uses and abuses, so it is worth considering each in detail.

Electrocochleogram (ECochG)

(Synonyms: ECoG, transtympanic electrocochleography)

Here an electrode is inserted transtympanically on to the middle ear promontory by an otologist with the aid of microscopic vision. In adults the electrode can be inserted without an anaesthetic as it is no more painful than a venepuncture. A local anaesthetic can be used but in children it is preferable to give a general anaesthetic.

It is possible to make similar but smaller recordings from electrodes placed on the skin of the external auditory canal near the tympanic membrane. This has the advantage of not requiring a doctor to insert the electrode and is less painful. The responses are smaller but usually adequate.

The ECochG responses are made up of three components which can be separated out by computer subtraction methods (*Figure AVII.1*):

(1) The compound action potential (CAP): This is the electrical response in the auditory nerve and is useful for determining thresholds. It is also considered by some to be of potential value in the diagnosis of auditory nerve pathology, such as acoustic neuroma or multiple sclerosis.
(2) Cochlear microphonics (CM): This is the hair cell response which in theory could be of value in diagnosing hair cell pathology but this is not yet practical because artefacts, similar to the CM, cannot be eliminated.
(3) Summating potential (SP): This is of uncertain origin and at present of no practical value though there are claims that abnormalities are present when there is endolymphatic hydrops (see p. 169).

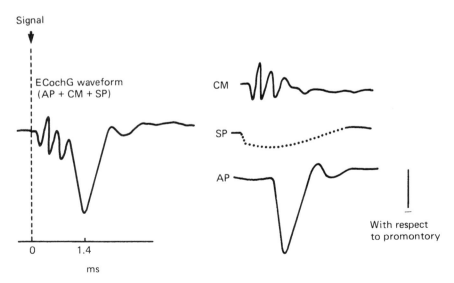

Figure AVII.1 Typical electrocochleographic response, with its three component responses: CM = cochlear microphonics; SP = summating potential; AP = action potential

Advantages

- Records close to the origin of the electrical response, giving quick and accurate recordings.
- Does not require masking of the non-test ear.

Disadvantages

- Requires a general anaesthetic in children and may require a local anaesthetic or sedation in adults.
- Poor reliability in assessing thresholds at or below 500 Hz.

Auditory brain stem response (ABR)

[Synonyms: brain stem evoked response (BSER)]

ABR is the preferred method to detect neuro-otological pathology. It can also be used to determine thresholds. Two active electrodes are required and these are usually placed on the vertex and on the ear lobe. In attempting to identify neurological disease, broad tonal clicks are used in order to achieve maximal stimulation so that abnormal latencies and absent waveforms are more readily apparent. In assessing thresholds, tone pips or filtered clicks are used.

The nomenclature used in naming the peaks in the ABR response varies but the most common method is to name the positive responses (with respect to the vertex) waves I to VI (*Figure AVII.2*). The levels in the auditory pathway at which these are said to originate are: I, VIIIth nerve at exit from cochlea; II, VIIIth nerve at entry to brain stem; III, cochlear nucleus; IV, superior olivary complex; V, lateral lemniscus and inferior colliculus.

Sedation or a general anaesthetic is usually required in children to keep them sufficiently still for the length of time it takes to assess thresholds. Many different medications have been used, none being so outstandingly successful that it has been accepted by all. What is needed is sedation rather than anaesthesia, so an oral dose of a tranquillizer such as a benzodiazepine, for example diazepam (Valium), is all that is often necessary. If such a premedication is insufficient then it can be 'topped up' with an intravenous injection. Some otologists prefer to use intramuscular ketamine.

Advantages

- It is not an invasive procedure.
- It is not affected by sedation.

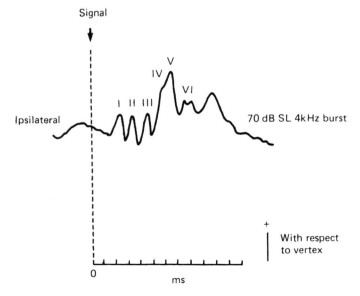

Figure AVII.2 Typical auditory brain stem responses

Disadvantages

- It needs a co-operative or sedated patient.
- For threshold assessments, the responses are small and therefore difficult to interpret.
- The thresholds are not so accurate at low as opposed to high frequencies.

Cortical evoked potentials

(Synonyms: cortical responses, slow vertex electric responses)

Cortical evoked responses were the first of the three main types of ERA to be used clinically and they still have a considerable role in determining thresholds but are of minimal value in detecting neuro-otological pathology.

The electrodes are usually sited on the vertex and the ear lobe and because of the long response latency, long tone-bursts are used. The waveform that is recorded (*Figure AVII.3*) has two positive (P1, P2) and two negative peaks (N1, N2). The N1 and P2 peaks are considered to reliably indicate a response.

Advantage

- This is the best of the three methods to determine thresholds across all the frequencies.

Disadvantage

- It is affected by sedation and is therefore not commonly used in children.

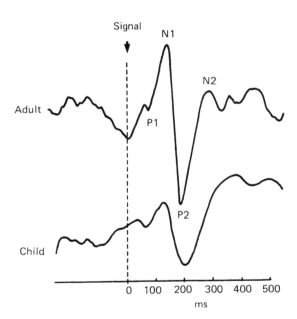

Figure AVII.3 Typical cortical evoked response

■ Conclusions

- Electric response audiometry (ERA) is not an objective test as the tester has to interpret the tracings.

- Considerable experience is required before the tracings can be readily interpreted.
- As with all forms of audiometry, the test

environment, calibration and masking of the non-test ear are extremely important if reliable thresholds are to be obtained.

- It is always preferable to assess pure tone thresholds by conventional means if at all possible.
- Cortical evoked potentials is the technique of choice in assessing pure tone thresholds when sedation is not required as is most often the case with adults.
- When sedation is required to keep the subject inactive, and this is frequently necessary in children, auditory brain stem response (ABR) or electrocochleography (ECochG) are the techniques of choice in assessing pure tone thresholds, but these techniques are less reliable at low frequencies than cortical responses.

- It is important to assess two or more thresholds by ERA as the correlation at a single frequency between the ERA and the pure tone thresholds can be poor.
- In attempting to detect neurological pathology, such as endolymphatic hydrops and acoustic neuroma, ABR and ECochG are the techniques of choice.

Further reading

Gelfand, S.A. (1997b). Physiological methods in audiology. Chap. 11. In *Essentials of Audiology.* Thieme Verlag, New York.

Lutman, M.E. (1997). Diagnostic audiometry. In *Adult Audiology*, Vol. 2, Scott-Brown's Otolaryngology. Butterworth-Heinemann, Oxford.

Appendix VIII

Oto-acoustic emissions

Sensitive microphones can record sounds being emitted from a normal ear. Such spontaneous oto-acoustic emissions (OAE) or cochlear echoes are thought to originate from the noise created by movement of the outer hair cells in the cochlea. If the ear is stimulated by noise, such as a click or tone-burst, this evokes oto-acoustic emissions which can be more easily recorded when present. Such evoked oto-acoustic emissions (EOAE) cannot be recorded if there is a conductive impairment or a sensorineural impairment.

Testing does not require patient co-operation and is performed with a two-channel ear tip, one channel to present the sound and the other to record sound. A transient click is presented and this is recorded on a tracing followed a few milliseconds later by the cochlear echo if present. As with electric response audiometry, multiple recordings allow the tracing to be classified by averaging of the responses.

Clinical applicability

Measuring oto-acoustic emissions is a relatively new technique which has already found a role in the screening of neonates. Its use in adults is as yet limited, but it could be used in patients with exaggerated thresholds and might be of value in investigating inner and outer hair cell function.

Appendix IX

Positional testing

Several different methods have been described, no one being more correct than the other. For most otologists a simple screening method is all that is necessary to decide whether positional factors are present and if they are then to decide the relative contributions of head position in relation to gravity and neck movements.

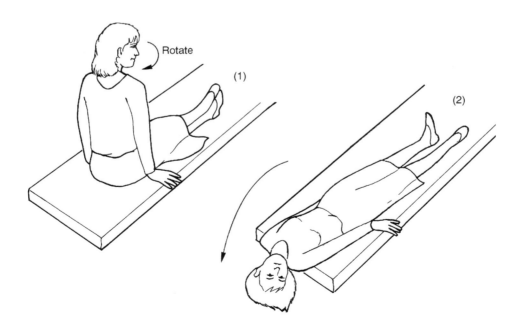

Rotate

(1)

(2)

Figure AIX.1 Hallpike manoevre

Neck movements

The patient is kept seated and the examiner goes behind and holds the patient's head with their hands. The head is gently moved forwards and sideways to assess the mobility of the cervical spine. If no symptoms are provoked then the neck is gradually rotated to one side and the neck extended. This is repeated to the other side. If dizziness is provoked the assumption is that cervical osteoarthritis is causing ischaemia due to vertebral artery compression.

Head position

Having confirmed that neck movements do not provoke symptoms the next question is whether the head position with respect to gravity will do this, the diagnosis being looked for being benign positional paroxysmal vertigo (see p. 166). Several methods have being described, the classical one being the Hallpike manoeuvre (*Figure AIX.1*). The patient is sat with their legs on a couch. The head is held by the examiner, rotated to one side, and the patient instructed to keep their eyes open with their gaze fixed on the examiner's eyes. They are then lain supine with the head hanging and still rotated over the end of the couch. Nystagmus is looked for and the patient asked if they have rotational vertigo. If symptom-free after 30 seconds they are then moved back to the sitting position and nystagmus and symptoms looked for again. Thereafter, if symptom-free, the procedure is repeated with the head turned to the other side.

References

Adams, D.A. (1997a). The causes of deafness. In *Paediatric Otolaryngology*, Vol. 6, Chap. 4. Scott-Brown's Otolaryngology, 6th Edition. Butterworth-Heinemann, Oxford.

Adams, D.A. (1997b). Management of the hearing impaired child. *Paediatric Otolaryngology*, Vol. 6, Chap. 10, Scott-Brown's Otolaryngology, 6th Edition. Butterworth-Heinemann, Oxford.

Alberti, P.W. (1981). Non-organic hearing loss in adults. In *Audiology and Audiological Medicine* (H.A. Beagley, ed.), 910–931. University Press, New York.

Alford, B.R. (1972). Ménière's disease. Criteria for diagnosis and evaluation of therapy for reporting. *Trans. Am. Acad. Ophthalmol. Otol.*, **74**, 1462–1464.

Appelman, C.L.M., Claessen, J.Q.P.J., Touw-Otten, F.W.M.M., Hordijk, G.J. and de Melker, R.A. (1991). Co-amoxiclav in recurrent acute otitis media: placebo controlled study. *Br. Med. J.*, **303**, 1450–1452.

Austin, D.F. (1978). Sound conduction of the diseased ear. *J. Laryngol. Otol*, **92**, 367–393.

Barber, H.O. (1975). Diagnostic techniques in vertigo. *J. Laryngol. and Otol.*, **92**, 367–393.

Benyon, G.J. (1997). A review of management of benign paroxysmal positional vertigo by exercise therapy and by repositioning manoeuvres. *Br. J. of Aud.*, **31**, 11–26.

Berliner, K.I., Doyle, K.J. and Goldenberg, R.A. (1996). Reporting operative hearing results in stapes surgery: does choice of outcome measure make a difference? *Am. J. Otol.*, **17**, 214–220.

Booth, J.B. (1997) Sudden and fluctuated sensorineural hearing. In *Otology*, Vol. 3, Chap. 17. Scott-Brown's Otolaryngology, 6th Edition. Butterworth-Heinemann, Oxford.

Bretlau, P., Salomon, G. and Johnsen, N.J. (1989). Otospongiosis and sodium fluoride. A clinical double-blind, placebo-controlled study on sodium fluoride treatment in otospongiosis. *Am. J. Otol.*, **10**, (1), 20–22.

British Association of Otolaryngologists and the British Society of Audiology (1983). Method for assessment of hearing disability. *Br. J. of Aud.*, **17**, 203–212.

British Society of Audiology (1981). Recommended procedures for pure-tone audiometry using a manually operated instrument. *Br. J. Audiol.*, **15**, 213–216.

British Society of Audiology (1985). Technical note: Re-

commended procedure for pure-tone bone-conduction audiometry without masking using a manually operated instrument. *Br. J. Audiol.*, **19**, 281–282.

British Society of Audiology (1986). Technical note: Recommendations for masking in pure tone threshold audiometry. *Br. J. Audiol.*, **20**, 307–314.

Browning, G.G. (1984). The unsafeness of 'safe' ears. *J. Laryngol. Otol.*, **98**, 23–26.

Browning, G.G. (1987). Guest editorial: Is there still a role for tuning-fork tests? *Br. J. of Aud.*, **21**, 161–163.

Browning, G.G. (1988). Medical management of active chronic otitis media: A controlled study. *J. Laryngol. Otol*, **102**, 491–495.

Browning, G.G. (1997a). Aetiopathology of inflammatory conditions of the external and middle ear. In *Otology*, Vol. 3, Chap. 2, Scott-Brown's Otolaryngology, 6th Edition, Butterworth-Heinemann, Oxford.

Browning, G.G. (1997b). Do patients and surgeons agree? The Gordon Smyth Memorial Lecture. *Clin. Otolaryngol*, **22**, 485–496.

Browning, G.G. and Davis, A. (1983). Clinical characterization of the hearing of the adult British population. *Advances in Oto-Rhino-Laryngol.*, **31**, 217–223.

Browning, G.G. and Gatehouse, S. (1983). Hearing in chronic otitis media. *Clin. Otolaryngol.*, **8**, 368.

Browning, G.G. and Gatehouse, S. (1984). Sensorineural hearing loss in stapedial otosclerosis. *Ann. Otol., Rhinol. Laryngol.*, **93**, 13–16.

Browning, G.G. and Gatehouse, S. (1992). The prevalence of middle ear disease in the adult British population. *Clin. Otolaryngol.*, **17**, 317–321.

Browning, G.G. and Gatehouse, S. (1994). Estimation of the benefit of bone-anchored hearing aids. *Ann. Otol. Rhino. Laryngol.*, **103**, (11), 872–878.

Browning, G.G. and Swan, I.R.C. (1982). Hearing loss in minor head surgery. *Arch. Otolaryngol.*, **108**, 474–477.

Browning, G.G. and Swan, I.R.C. (1988). Sensitivity and specificity of the Rinne tuning fork test. *Br. Med. J.*, **297**, 1381–1382.

Browning, G.G., Gatehouse, S. and Calder, I.T. (1988). Medical management of active chronic otitis media: A controlled study. *J. Laryngol. Otol.*, **102**, 491–495.

Browning, G.G., Picozzi, G.L., Calder, I.T. and Sweeney, G.

(1983). Controlled trial of medical management of active chronic otitis media. BMJ, **28**, (7) 1024.

Browning, G.G., Swan, I.R.C. and Chew, K.K. (1989). Clinical role of informal tests of hearing. *J. Laryngol. Otol.*, **103**, 7–11.

Browning, G.G., Swan, I.R.C. and Gatehouse, S. (1982). Hearing loss in minor head injury. *Arch. Otolaryngol.*, **108**, 474–477.

Browning, G.G., Swan, I.R.C. and Gatehouse, S. (1985). The doubtful nature of tympanometry in the diagnosis of otosclerosis. *J. Laryngol. Otol.*, **99**, 545–547.

Byrne, D. and Dillon, H. (1986). The National Acoustic Laboratories (NAL) new procedure for selecting the gain and frequency response of a hearing aid. *Ear Hear.*, **7**, 257–265.

Carhart, R. (1950). Clinical application of bone conduction audiometry. *Arch. Otolaryngol.*, **51**, 798–808.

Casselbrant, M.L., Kaleida, P.H., Rockette, H.E., Paradise, J.L., Bluestone, C.D., Kurs-Lasky, M., Nozza, R.J. and Wald, E.R. (1992). Efficacy of antimicrobial prophylaxis and of tympanostomy tube insertion for prevention of recurrent acute otitis media: results of a randomized clinical trial. *Ped. Infect. Dis. J.*, **11**, 278–286.

Cawthorne–Cooksey regime of head exercises (1997). In *Otology*, Vol. 3, Appendix 12.1, p. 3/12/27, Scott-Brown's Otolaryngology, 6th Edition. Butterworth-Heinemann, Oxford.

Chandrasekhar, S.S., Brackmann, D.E. and Devgan, K.K. (1995). Utility of auditory brainstem response audiometry in diagnosis of acoustic neuromas. *Am. J. Otol.*, **16**, 63–67.

Ciuffetti, G., Scardazza, A., Serafini, G., Lombardini, R., Mannarino, E. and Simoncelli, C. (1991). Whole-blood filterability in sudden deafness. *Laryngoscope*, **101**, 65–67.

Coles, R.R.A. (1982). Non-organic hearing loss. In *Otology* (A.G. Gibb and M.F.W. Smith, eds), pp. 150–176. Butterworths, Oxford.

Coles, R.R.A. (1996). In *Tinnitus.*, Vol. 2, Chap. 18. (S.D.G. Stephens, ed. A.G. Kerr, gen. ed.). Scott-Brown's Otolaryngology, 6th Edition. Butterworth-Heinemann, Oxford.

Coles, R.R.A. and Mason, S.M. (1984). The results of cortical electric response audiometry in medico-legal investigations. *Br. J. Audiol.*, **18**, 71–78.

Commins, D.J. and Nedzelski, J.M. (1996). Current diagnostics and office practice. Topical drugs in the treatment of Meniere's disease. *Cur. Opin. Otolaryngol. Head Neck Surg.*, **4**, 319–323.

Coles, R.R.A. and Priede, V.M. (1977). Derivations of formulae for masking of the non-test ear in speech audiometry. *Institute of Sound and Vibration Research Memorandum No. 448*. 1977 Revision, Southampton.

Committee on Conservation of Hearing of the American Academy of Ophthalmology and Otolaryngology (1965). Standard classification for surgery of chronic ear infection. *Arch. Otolaryngol.*, **81**, 204–205.

Committee on Hearing and Equilibrium guidelines for the evaluation of results of treatment of conductive hearing loss (1995). *Otolaryngol. Head Neck Surg.*, **113**, 186–187.

Crowley, H. and Kaufman, R.S. (1966). The Rinne tuning fork test. *Arch. Otolaryngol.*, **84**, 406–408.

Culford, S.A. (1997). Acoustic Immitance Assessment, Chap. 7. In *Essentials of Audiology* (S.A. Culford, ed.). Thieme Verlag, New York.

Daly, K.A. (1991). Epidemiology of otitis media. *Otolaryngol. Clin. Nth. Am.*, **24**, 775–786.

Davis, A.C. (1989). The prevalence of hearing impairment and reported hearing disability among adults in Great Britain. *Inter. J. Epidem.*, **18**, 911–917.

Davis, A.C. (1995). *Hearing in Adults*. Whurr, London.

Davis, A.G. (1997). Epidemiology. In *Adult Audiology*, Vol. 2, Chap. 3, Scott-Brown's Otolaryngology, 6th Edition. Butterworth-Heinemann, Oxford.

Davis, A., Bamford J., Wilson, I., Ramkalavan, T., Forshaw, M. and Wright, S. (1997). A critical review of the role of neonatal screening in the detection of congenital hearing impairment. Report submitted to Department of Health.

Davis, H. (1984). Slow cortical evoked potential. *Acta Otolaryngologia* (Supplement) **206**, 128–134.

Day, G.A., Browning, G.G. and Gatehouse S. (1988). Benefit from binaural hearing aids in individuals with a severe hearing impairment. *Br. J. Audiol.*, **22**, 273–277.

Del Mar C., Glaszion P. and Hayem M. (1997). Are antibiotics indicated as initial treatment for children with acute otitis media? A meta analysis. *BMJ*, **314**, 1526–1529.

Dempster, J.H., Browning, G.G. and Gatehouse, S. (1993). A randomized study of the surgical management of children with persistent otitis media with effusion associated with a hearing impairment. *J. Laryngol. Otol.*, **107**, 284–289.

Dempster, J.H. and MacKenzie, K. (1991). Tympanometry in the detection of hearing impairments associated with otitis media with effusion. *Clin. Otolaryngol.*, **16**, 157–159.

Dempster, J.H. and Swan, I.R.C. (1988). The management of otitis media with effusion in adults. *Clin. Otolaryngol.*, **13**, 197–199.

De Michele, A.M. and Ruth, R.A. (1996). The diagnostic use of auditory brainstem response and evoked otoacoustic emissions in the era of magnetic resonance imaging. *Cur. Opin. Otolaryngol. Head Neck Surg.*, **4**, 356–359.

Department of Health and Human Services (1994). Managing otitis media with effusion in young children. *Quick Reference Guide for Clinicians*, **12**.

Doyle, P.S., Anderson, D.W. and Pijl, S. (1984). The tuning fork – an essential instrument in otological practice. *J. Otolaryngol.*, **13**, 83–86.

Effective Health Care Bulletin (1992). The treatment of persistent glue ear in children. *Effect. Health Care*, **4**.

Erlandsson, S., Ringdahl, A., Hutchins, T. and Carlsson, S.G. (1987). Treatment of tinnitus: a controlled comparison of masking and placebo. *Brit. J. Audiol.*, **21**, 37–44.

Evans, D.G.R. and Ramsden, R.T. (1995). Neurofibromatosis type 2. In *Recent Adv. Otolaryngol.*, **7**, 181–189.

Farmer, J.C. and Gillespie, C.A. (1997). Pathophysiology of the ear and nasal sinuses in flight and diving. In *Basic Sciences*, Vol. I, Chap. 7, Scott-Brown's Otolaryngology, 6th Edition. Butterworth-Heinemann, Oxford.

Finitzo, T., Friel-Patti, S., Chinn, K. and Brown, O. (1992). Tympanometry and otoscopy prior to myringotomy: issues in diagnosis of otitis media. *Inter. J. Ped. Otorhinolaryngol.*, **24**, 101–110.

Fischer, A.J.B.M., Verhagen, W.I.M. and Huygen, P.L.M. (1997). Whiplash injury. A clinical review with emphasis on neuro-otological aspects. *Rev. Clin. Otolaryngol*, **22**, 192–201.

Fortnum, H. and Davis, A. (1993). Hearing impairment in children after bacterial meningitis: incidence and resource implication. *Br. J. Audiol.*, **94**, 113–117.

Fortnum, H. and Davis, A. (1997). Epidemiology of permanent childhood hearing impairment in Trent Region. 1985–93. *Br. J. Audiol.*, **31**, 409–446.

Fraser, G.R. (1976). *The Causes of Profound Deafness in Children*. Baillière Tindall, London.

Gaihede, M. (1998). High negative middle ear pressure explained by tympanometric artefacts in secretory otitis media. *Recent Advances in Otitis Media* (M. Tos, J. Thomsen and V. Balle, eds). Kugler Publications, Amsterdam.

Gatehouse, S. (1983). Central auditory function following a severe head injury. *Clin. Otolaryngol.*, **9**, 129–130.

Gatehouse, S.G. (1997). Hearing aids. In *Audiology*, Vol. 2, Scott-Brown's Otolaryngology, 6th Edition, Butterworth-Heinemann, Oxford.

Gatehouse, S.G. (1998). The Glasgow Hearing Aid Benefit Profile in a client centred approach and disability, discharge and hearing aid benefit. *J. Am. Acad. Audiol.*, In press.

Gatehouse, S. and Browning, G.G. (1982). A re-examination of the Carhart effect. *Br. J. Audiol.*, **16**, 215–220.

Gatehouse, S. and Browning, G.G. (1990) The output characteristics of an implanted bone conduction prosthesis. *Clin. Otolaryngol.*, **15**, 503–513

Gates, G.A., Cobb, J.L., D'Agostino, R.B., and Wolf, P.A. (1993). The relation of hearing in the elderly to the presence of cardiovascular disease and cardiovascular risk factors. *Arch. Otolaryngol. Head Neck. Surg.*, **119**, 156–161.

Gelfand, S.A. (1977). Clinical precision of the Rinne test. *Acta Otolaryngol.*, **84**, 480–487.

Gelfand, S.A. (1997a). Acoustic Immitance Assessment, Chap. 7. In *Essentials of Audiology*. Thieme Verlag, New York.

Gelfand, S.A. (1997b). Physiological methods in audiology. *Essentials of Audiology*. Thieme Verlag, New York.

General Household Survey (1983). The prevalence of tinnitus 1981. OPCS Monitor GHS 83/1. Office of Population Censuses and Surveys, London.

Gibbin, K.P. (1997). Cochlear implantation in children. In *Paediatric Otolaryngology*, Vol. 6, Chap. 11. Scott-Brown's Otolaryngology. Butterworth-Heinemann, Oxford.

Giles, M. (1997). Severe mixed hearing impairments. *MD Thesis*, University of Auckland.

Giles, M., Browning, G.G. and Gatehouse, S. (1996). Problems in assessing the audiogram in patients with severe hearing impairment. *J. Laryngol. Otol.*, **110**, 727–731.

Ginsberg, I.A., Hoffman, S.R., White, T.P. and Stinzano, G.D. (1978). Stapedectomy – in depth analysis of 2405 cases. *Laryngoscope*, **88**, 1999–2016.

Glasgold, A. and Altman, R. (1965). The effects of stapes surgery on tinnitus in otosclerosis. *Laryngoscope*, **76**, 1524–1532.

Glorig, A. and Gallo, R. (1962). Comments on sensorineural hearing loss in otosclerosis. In *Otosclerosis*, pp. 63–78. Little Brown & Co., Boston, M.A.

Golabek, W. and Stephens, S.D.G. (1979). Some tuning fork tests revisited. *Clin. Otolaryngol.*, **4**, 421–430.

Goldenberg, R.A., and Berliner, K.I. (1995). Reporting operative hearing results: does choice of outcome measure make a difference? *Am. J. Otol.*, **16**, 128–135.

Gordon, M.L. and Cohen, N.L. (1995). Efficacy of auditory brainstem response as a screening test for small acoustic neuromas. *Am. J. of Otol.*, **16**, 136–139.

Gunderson, T. (1973). Sensorineural hearing loss in otosclerosis. *Scand. Audiol.*, **4**, 43–51.

Hakansson, B., Liden, G., Tjellstrom A., Ringdahl, A., Jacobsson, M., Carlsson, P. and Erlandson, B.J. (1990). Ten years of experience with the Swedish bone-anchored hearing system. *Ann. Otorhinolaryngol.*, **99**, (10, 2), Suppl.151, 1–16.

Hall, S.J., Kerr, A.G., Varghese, M., Milliken, T.G. and Patterson, C.C. (1985). Deafness in hypothyroidism. ORS abstracts, Birmingham, April 1985. *Clin. Otolaryngol.*, **10**, 292.

Hall, S.J., McGuigan, J.A. and Rocks, M.J. (1991). Red blood cell deformability in sudden sensorineural deafness: another aetiology? *Clin. Otolaryngol.* **16**, 3–7.

Harrison, M.S. and Ozsahinoglu, C. (1972). Positional vertigo: aetiology and clinical significance. *Brain*, **95**, 369–372.

Haughton, P.M. (1977). Validity of tympanometry for middle ear effusions. *Arch. Otolaryngol.*, **103**, 505–513.

Hinchcliffe, R. (1955). Sound hazards and their control. Unpublished dissertation. University of Manchester.

Hinchcliffe, R. (1981). Clinical tests of auditory function in the adult and the school child. In *Audiology and Audiological Medicine*, pp. 319–364. Edited by Beagley, H. A. Oxford University Press, Oxford.

House, P.R. (1981). Personality of the tinnitus patient. In *Tinnitus. Ciba Foundation Symposium 85*, pp. 204–212. Pitman, London.

House, J.W. and Brackman, D.E. (1981). Tinnitus: surgical treatment. In *Tinnitus. Ciba Foundation Symposium 85*, pp. 204–212. Pitman, London.

International Standards Organization (1964). Standard reference zero for the calibration of pure tone audiometers. ISO Recommendation R389. American National Standards Institute, Inc., New York.

Jaffe, B.R. (1981). Are water and tympanotomy tubes compatible? *Laryngoscope*, **91**, 563–564.

Jastreboff, P.J. and Hazell, J.W.P. (1993). A neurophysiological approach to tinnitus: clinical implications. *Br. J. Audiol.*, **27**, 7–17.

Jerger, J., Anthony, L., Jerger, S. and Mauldin, L. (1974). Studies in impedance audiometry. III Middle ear disorders, *Arch. Otolaryngol.*, **99**, 165–171.

Jerger, J., Jerger, S. and Mauldin, L. (1972). Studies in impedance audiometry. I Normal and sensorineural ears. *Arch. Otolaryngol.*, **96**, 513–523.

Jerger, J. and Northern, J.L. (1980). *Clinical Impedance Audiometry*, 2nd Edition. American Electromedics Corporation, Acton, MA.

Jones, N.S. (1997). Hyperlipidaemia and hearing loss. *MD Thesis*. University of London.

Kazanas, S.G. and Maw, A.R. (1994). Tympanometry, stapedius reflex and hearing impairment in children with otitis media with effusion. *Acta Otolaryngol. (Stockh)*, **114**, 410–414.

Kerr, A.G. and Adams, D.A. (1983). Congenital syphilitic deafness – a long-term follow-up. *Adv. Oto-Rhino-Laryngol.*, **31**, 247–252.

King, P.F., Coles, R.R.A., Lutman, M.E. and Robinson, D.W. (1992). *Assessment of Hearing Disability.* Guidelines for medico-legal practice. Whurr, London.

Kraus, E.M. and Dubois, P.J. (1979). Tomography of the

vestibular aqueduct in ear disease. *Arch. Otolaryngol.*, **105**, 91–98.

Lancet Editorial (1984). Vestibular function in microgravity, **ii**, 561.

Lancet Editorial (1987). Hearing problems in elderly people: implications for services. *Lancet*, 1181–1182.

Lerner, A.M., Cone, A.L., Jansen, W., Reyes, M.P., Blair, D.C., Wright, G.E. and Lorber, R.R. (1983). Randomised, controlled trial of the comparative efficacy, auditory toxicity, and nephrotoxicity of tobramycin and Netilmicin. *Lancet*, **i**, 1123–1125.

Lutman, M.E. (1984). The relationship between acoustic reflex threshold and air–bone gap. *Br. J. Audiol.*, **18**, 223–229.

Lutman, M.E. (1986). Acoustic impedance audiometry. In *Physics in Medicine and Biology Encyclopaedia* (T.E. McAinsh, ed.). Pergamon Press, Oxford.

Lutman, M.E. (1997). Diagnostic audiometry. In *Adult Audiology*, Vol. 2, Scott-Brown's Otolaryngology. Butterworth-Heinemann, Oxford.

McClymont, L.G. and Browning, G.G. (1991). Characterization of severely and profoundly hearing impaired adults attending an audiology clinic. *J. Laryngol. Otol.*, **105**, 534–538.

McCormick, B. (1997). Screening and surveillance for hearing impairment in pre-school children, In *Paediatric Otolaryngology.* Vol. 6, Chap. 6, Scott-Brown's Otolaryngology, 6th Edition. Butterworth-Heinemann, Oxford.

McFadden, D. (1982). In *Tinnitus. Facts, Theories and Treatments*, pp. 89–116. Working Groups 89 Committee on Hearing. National Research Council. National Academy Press, Washington DC.

McGarry, G.W. and Swan I.R.C. (1992). Endoscopic photographic comparison of drug delivery by ear-drops and by aerosol spray. *Clin. Otolaryngol.*, **17**, 359–360.

McKee, G.J. and Stephens, S.D.G. (1992). An investigation of normally hearing subjects with tinnitus. *Audiol.*, **31**, 313–317.

Martin, F.W. and Colman, B.H. (1980). Tinnitus: a double-blind crossover controlled trial to evauate the use of lignocaine. *Clin. Otolaryngol.*, **5**, 3–11.

Maw, A.R. and Herod, F. (1986). Otoscopic, impedance and audiometric findings in glue ear treated by adenoidectomy and tonsillectomy: a prospective randomised study. *Lancet*, **1**, 1399–1402.

Medical Research Council, Institute of Hearing Research (1981). Epidemiology of tinnitus. In *Tinnitus. Ciba Foundation Symposium 85*, pp. 16–34.

Medical Research Council, Institute of Hearing Research (1984). Epidemiology of tinnitus (1) prevalence, (2) demographic and clinical features. *J. Laryngol. Otol.*, (Suppl.) 9, 7–15 and 195–202.

Medical Research Council Multi-centre Target report (1998). The role of tympanometry in predicting an associated hearing impairment in children with otitis media with effusion. *Clin. Otolaryngol.* In press.

Moeller, H., Browning, G.G. and Gatehouse, S. (1997). Hearing in patients with Paget's disease. *Clin. Otolaryngol.* In press.

Montandon, P.B. and Hausler, R. (1984). Relevance of otopathological findings in the treatment of dizzy patients. *Ann. Otol., Rhinol. Laryngol.*, (Suppl.) **93**, 112, 12–14.

Mylanus, E.A.M., Snik, A.FM., Cremers, C.W.R.J., Jarritsma, F.F. and Verschuure H. (1994). Audiological results of the bone-anchored hearing aid HC200: Multicenter results. *Ann. Otol. Rhino. Laryngol.*, **103**, 368–374.

Normura, Y., Okund, T. and Kawabata, I. (1983). The round window membrane. In *Mod. Perspec. Otolol. Ad. Oto-Rhino-Laryngol.*, **31**, 50–58.

Norre, M.E. and Beckers, A. (1987). Exercise treatment for paroxysmal positional vertigo: Comparison of two types of exercises. *Arch. Otolaryngol.*, **244**, 291–294.

Nunez, D. and Browning, G.G. (1989). The risks of developing an otogenic intracranial abscess. *J. Laryngol. Otol.*, **104**, 468–472.

Ohinata, Y., Makimoto, K., Kawakami, M., Haginomori, S.I., Araki, M. and Takahashi, H. (1994). Blood viscosity and plasma viscosity in patients with sudden deafness. *Acta Otolaryngol (Stockh)*, **114**, 601–607.

Orchik, D.J. (1978). Tympanometry as a predictor of middle ear fluid. *Arch. Otolaryngol.*, **104**, 4–6.

Parving, A., Parving, H.H. and Lyngs, O.E. (1983). Hearing sensitivity in patients with myxoedema before and after treatment with L-thyroxine. *Acta Otolaryngologica*, **95**, 315–321.

Picozzi, G.L., Browning, G.G. and Calder, I.T. (1983). Controlled trial of gentamicin and hydrocortisone ear drops in the treatment of active chronic otitis media. *Clin. Otolaryngol.*, **8**, 36.

Plantenga, J.F. (1983). Endolymfatishche hydrops by ziekte van Ménière. Rodopi, Amsterdam.

Plantenga, J.F. and Browning, G.G. (1979). The vestibular aqueduct and endolymphatic sac and duct in endolymphatic hydrops. *Arch. Otolaryngol.*, **105**, 546–552.

Robinson, D.W. and Dadson, R.S. (1957). Threshold of hearing and equal-loudness relations for pure-tone, and the loudness function. *J. Acoust. Soc. Am.*, **29**, 1284–1288.

Robinson, D.W. and Shipton, M.S. (1973). Tables for the estimation of noise-induced hearing loss. *National Physical Laboratory Report Ac 61*.

Robinson, D.W. and Shipton, M.S. (1977). Tables for the estimation of noise induced hearing loss. *National Physics Laboratory Acoustics Report AC 61*. National Physics Laboratory, Teddington.

Saeed, S.R. and Brookes, G.B. (1993). The use of clostridium botulinum toxin in palatal myoclonus: a preliminary report. *J. Laryngol. Otol.*, **107**, 208–210.

Sakai, M. (1994). Editorial: Proposal of a guideline in reporting hearing results in middle ear and mastoid surgery. *Am. J. Otol.*, **15**, (3), 291–293.

Sataloff, J., Farb, S., Menduke, H. and Vassalo, L. (1964). Sensorineural hearing loss in otosclerosis. *Trans. Am. Acad. Ophthalmol. Otorhinolaryngol.*, **65**, 243–248.

Schuknecht, H.F. (1969). Cupulolithiasis. *Arch. Otolaryngol.*, **90**, 765–778.

Schuknecht, H.F. (1974). *Pathology of the Ear.* Harvard University Press, Boston, MA.

Shaw, E.A.G. (1974). Transformation of sound pressure level from the free field to the ear drum in the horizontal plane. *J. Acoust. Soc. Am.*, **56**, 1848–1561.

Shepard, N.T. and Telian S.A. (1996). *Practical Management of the Balance Disorder Patient*. Singular Publishing Group, San Diego, London.

Shimoda, T. and Limm, D.J. (1971). The fibre arrangement of the human tympanic membrane. A scanning electron microscopic observation. *Ann. Otolaryngol.*, **80**, 210–217.

Singh, B. and Maharaj, T.J. (1993). Radical mastoidectomy: its place in otitic intracranial complications. *J. Laryngol. Otol.*, **107**, 1113–1118.

Sirimanna T., Stephens, D. and Board, T. (1996). Tinnitus and audioscan notches. *J. Audiol. Med.*, **5**, 1, 38–48.

Smyth, G.D.L. (1985). Results of middle ear reconstruction: do patients and surgeons agree? *Am. J. Otol.* **6**, 276–279.

Snik, A.F.M., Jorritsma, F.F., Cremers, C.W.R.J., Beynon, A.J. and van den Berge, N.W. (1992). The super-bass bone-anchored hearing aid compared to conventional hearing aids. Audiological results and the patients' opinions. *Scand. Audiol.*, **21**, 157–161.

Snyder, J.M. (1973). Interaural attenuation characteristics in audiometry. *Laryngoscope*, **83**, 1847–1855.

Stahle, J. and Wilbrand, H. (1974). The vestibular aqueduct in patient with Ménière's disease. *Acta Otolaryngol.*, **78**, 36–48.

Stankiewicz, J.A. and Mowry, H.S. (1979). Clinical accuracy of tuning fork tests. *Laryngoscope*, **89**, 1956–1963.

Stevens, S.D.G. (1981). Clinical audiometry. In *Audiology and Audiological Medicine* H.A. Beagley, ed.), p. 374. Oxford University Press, Oxford.

Stool, S.E. and Flaherty, M.R. (1983). Algorithm for diagnosis of otitis media with effusion. *Annals of Otology, Rhinology and Laryngology*, **92**, Supplement 107, 6–7.

Summerfield, A.Q. and Marshall, D.H. (1995). Cochlear implantation in the UK, 1990–1994. Report by the MRC Institute of Hearing Research in the evaluation of the national cochlear implant programme. HMSO Publications, London.

Swan, I.R.C. (1984). Clinical aspects of hearing aid provision. *MD Thesis*, University of Glasgow.

Swan, I.R.C. (1989). Diagnostic vetting of individuals with asymmetric sensorineural hearing impairments. *J. Laryngol. Otol.*, **103**, 823–826.

Swan, I.R.C. (1997). Clinical tests of hearing and balance. In *Adult Audiology*, Vol. 2, Chap. 5, Scott-Brown's Otolaryngology, 6th Edition, Butterworth-Heinemann, Oxford.

Swan, I.R.C. and Browning, G.G. (1985). The whispered voice as a screening test for hearing loss. *J. R. Coll. Gen. Prac.*, **35**, 197.

Swan, I.R.C. and Browning, G.G. (1994). A prospective evaluation of direct referral to audiology departments for hearing aids. *J. Laryngol. Otol.*, **108**, 120–124.

Swan, I.R.C. and Gatehouse S. (1991). Clinical and financial audit of diagnostic protocols for lesions of the cerebellopontine angle. *BMJ.*, **302**, 701–704.

Swan, I.R.C. and Gatehouse, S. (1995). The value of routine in-the-ear measurement of hearing aid gain. *Brit. J. Audiol.*, **29**, 271–277.

Swan, I.R.C., Browning, G.G. and Gatehouse, S.G. (1983). Cross-over of the side of prescription of a hearing aid. *Clin. Otolaryngol.*, **8**, 136.

Tay, H.L., Ray, N., Ohri, R. and Frootko, N.J. (1995). Diabetes mellitus and hearing loss. *Clin. Otolaryngol.*, **20**, 130–134.

Tempest, W. and Bryan, M.E. (1981). Industrial hearing loss; compensation in the United Kingdom. In *Audiology and Audiological Medicine*, pp. 846–860. University Press, Oxford.

Thomsen, J., Brethan, P., Tos, M. and Johnsen, N.J. (1981). Placebo effect in surgery for Ménière's disease. A double-blind placebo-controlled study on endolymphatic sac shunt surgery. *Arch. Otolaryngol.*, **107**, 271–277.

Thomsen, J. and Vesterhauge, S. (1979). A critical evaluation of the glycerol test in Ménière's disease. *Advances in Oto-Rhino-Laryngol.*, **25**, 49–53.

Toner, J.G. and Smyth, G.D.L. (1993). Comparison of methods of evaluating hearing benefit of middle ear surgery. *J. Laryngol. Otol.* **107**, 4–5.

Tonndorf, J. (1972). Bone conduction. In *Foundations of Modern Auditory Theory.* Edited by Tobias, J.U. Academic Press, New York.

Tos, M. (1993). Approaches: Myringoplasty: Ossiculoplasty: Tympanoplasty. Vol. 1. In *Manual of Middle Ear Surgery.* Thieme Verlag, New York.

Tos, M., Hølm-Jensen, S., Sørensen, C.H. and Mogensen, C. (1982). Spontaneous course and frequency of secretory otitis in 4-year-old children *Arch. Otolaryngol.*, **108**, 4–9.

Tos, M., Stangerup, S-E. and Larsen, P. (1987). Dynamics of eardrum changes following secretory otitis: A prospective study. *Arch. Otolaryngol. Head Neck Surg.*, **113**, 380–385.

Travis, L.W. Stankiewicz, J.A. and Melvin, S.W. (1977). Impact trauma of the human temporal bone. *J. Trauma*, **17**, 761–766.

Tyler, R.S. and Conrad-Armes, D. (1982). Spontaneous acoustic cochlear emissions and sensorineural tinnitus. *Br. J. Audiol.*, **16**, 193–194.

Tyler, R.S. and Shum, D.J. (1995). *Assistive Devices for Persons with Hearing Impairment.* Allyn and Bacon, Boston.

van Buchem, F.L., Dunk, J.H.M. and van't Hof, M.A. (1981). Therapy of acute otitis media: myringotomy, antibiotics or neither? *Lancet*, **ii**, 884–887.

van Buchem, F.L., Peeters, M.F. and van't Hof, M.A. (1985). Acute otitis media: a new treatment strategy. *BMJ*, **290**, 1033–1037.

Vartiainen, E. and Vartiainen, J. (1996). The effect of drinking water fluoridation on the natural course of hearing in patients with otosclerosis. *Acta. Otolaryngol. (Stockh)*, **116**, 747–750.

Vesterager, V. (1997). Tinnitus – investigation and management. *Br. Med. J.*, **314**, 728–732.

Weiner, F.M. and Ross, D.A. (1946). The pressure distribution in the auditory canal in the progressive south field. *J. Acoust. Soc. Am.*, **18**, 401–408.

Wilson, W.R. and Woods, L.A. (1975). Accuracy of the Bing and Rinne tuning fork tests. *Arch. Otolaryngol*, **101**, 81–85.

Wormald, P.J. and Browning, G.G. (1996). *Otoscopy – a structured approach.* Arnold, London.

Zielhius, G.A., Rach, G.H., Van Den Bosch, A. and Van Den Broek P. (1990). The prevalence of otitis media with effusion: a critical review of the literature. *Clin. Otolaryngol.*, **15**, 283–288.

Zoller, M., Wilson, W.R. and Nadol, J.B. (1979). Treatment of syphilitic hearing loss: combined penicillin and steroid therapy in 29 patients. *Ann. Otol., Rhinol. Laryngol.*, **88**, 160–165.

Index